Cognitive Decline

Dr Craige Golding

These are the protocols and opinions of Dr Craige Golding.

Published by
The Golding Institute
65 Central Street
Houghton Estate
Johannesburg
2198

Written by Dr Craige Golding
Editing by Gwen Podbrey
Cover and layout by Dr Carel-Piet van Eeden

Cognitive Decline

This book is dedicated to every person touched by cognitive decline. Be it patient or loved one. May it bring hope and illumination to everyone.

"A man's real possession is his memory. In nothing else is he rich, in nothing else is he poor."

—ALEXANDER SMITH,
SCOTTISH POET (1829-1867)

Contents

TREATMENT OF COGNITIVE DECLINE 77

TREATING ALZHEIMER'S DISEASE 97

Introduction

Few diagnoses strike as much dismay in patients and their families as Alzheimer's disease. Although it does not properly belong in the category of "dread diseases", since it does not have the often rapid deleterious effect in individuals as, say, cancer, a heart attack (or, for that matter, Covid-19) and does not involve the distressing experiences of intensive care wards, oncological treatment or life support apparatus, it is automatically associated by many with the irrevocable decline of memory – and all that memory embodies: relationships, cognitive ability, awareness, dignity and, eventually, identity.

Yet this is no longer the case. Over the past decades, research into the condition has shown that it is largely preventable, with lifestyle modifications, and that treatment can not only significantly slow down the rate of cognitive decline in patients, but sometimes arrest it altogether or even reverse it enough to restore meaningful quality of life. There is plenty of hope and plenty of help available.

This book explains the pathology of Alzheimer's disease and cognitive decline, their causes, and their treatment. If you are reading this because you or a loved one has recently been diagnosed with it, we hope that it will provide you with the information you need to face the future with renewed confidence and courage.

Definition And Causes

WHAT IS COGNITIVE DECLINE?

Cognitive decline – or Alzheimer's disease – is the brain's protective response to three major metabolic and toxic disturbances. Like many other diseases, there are different forms – and severities – of it.

Classification of Alzheimer's Disease

Alzheimer's disease can be broadly categorised into five distinct types:

Type 1

This is caused by inflammation of the brain caused by infections, as well as by diabetes (diabetics are particularly prone to Alzheimer's disease later in life due to the effect of glucose on the brain), oral bacteria and inflammation of the gut. Inflammatory markers must be checked by the doctor and nutraceuticals such as circulin (an antibiotic consisting of a mixture of peptides) and Omega 3 prescribed to balance sugar and insulin resistance.

Type 2

This is caused by withdrawal of trophic support, resulting in decreased nerve growth factor and hormone decline. Neurotrophic support is needed in the form of proteins. Neurotrophins are critical to the structural integrity of adult neurons. They are essential for neural plasticity (the ability of neural networks in the brain to change through growth and re-organisation, such as making new connections and cortical remapping). Neural plasticity is essential for normal learning ability and all other functions supported by memory.

Type 3

This is caused by toxins. It can include what is known as *inhalational dementia*. This type can be caused by exposure to toxins such as divalent metals (mercury, aluminium, etc), as well as to biotoxins from *mould*, and the effects of certain proteins. These neurotoxic factors can also result in other neurodegenerative illnesses such as motor neuron disease, Parkinson's disease, multiple sclerosis, and many others. Tools to detect mould include oligo-lab, heavy metal testing, chronic inflammation tests and innate immune function testing.

Type 4

This is caused by vascular insufficiency, i.e., blockages in the carotid arteries which impair blood supply to the brain. The patient's medical history may show cardiac disease. Sleep insufficiency due to apnoea (a condition in which breathing repeatedly stops and starts during sleeping, typically with heavy snoring) is also a trigger of Type 4.

Type 5
Previous trauma to the brain (such as strokes, encephalitis, trauma caused by injury or multiple sclerosis) can trigger inflammation and cognitive decline.

Type 1.5
Combinations of the above types – a common occurrence. For example, glycotoxins such as smoke and divalent metals might cause brain inflammation and insulin resistance, which then leads to the loss of trophic support. Each combination of Alzheimer types includes a sequence of triggers and effects. These will inform the plurality of treatments which should be prescribed for a particular patient, since there is no single treatment which addresses all aspects of the disease in all patients.

Alzheimer's Disease vs Natural Age-Related Memory Decline
It is important to distinguish between natural, age-related memory decline and the condition of Alzheimer's disease.

Studies have found that people experience a natural, significant memory decline of 21% between the ages of 25 and

40. According to research conducted by American anti-ageing and metabolic medicine specialist Pamela Smith, this continues, so that by the ages of 70-79, memory decline is, on average, 43%. This can be considered part of the natural "wear and tear" process of the brain, and other organs, as we get older.

Alzheimer's Disease: What Happens Inside the Brain?

Alzheimer's disease, by contrast, is a systemic disorder of the brain – indeed, it is a type of molecular brain cancer, causing the build-up of **amyloid plaques** (abnormal proteins) in the spaces between nerve cells. The amyloids are produced in the bone marrow and can be deposited in any tissue or organ (usually the heart, kidneys, liver, spleen, nervous system, and digestive tract), as well as the brain. Amyloids are particularly dangerous, since it can take a long time before they cause any symptoms. Therefore, a patient is unaware of their condition until the amyloid plaque has already formed. In the brain, the plaques first develop in the areas associated with memory and other cognitive functions. It is crucial to remember that the formation of amyloid plaque is a **protective** response of the brain to the toxins and mould forming in it. The plaque is the **response to, or effect of,** the disease, not the **cause** of it. Treatment should therefore focus on the causes of the plaque.

Another primary characteristic of Alzheimer's disease is the development of neurofibrillary tangles of the brain tissue. These cause the twisting of protein threads of the nerve cells in the brain tissue. The result is a loss of memory and cognitive function. (Imagine the tangles which form in a mass of electrical cords and what would happen if you tried to plug one of them – for instance, the electrical cord of a headphone set, which was tangled up and distorted with many other cords – into an outlet. In all likelihood, the headphones would not work because the voltage flow through them would be obstructed by the tangles. The identical situation takes place when there are neurofibrillary tangles in the brain tissue: the nerve cells cannot receive or transmit the correct signals prompting memory and other cognitive functions requiring retention.)

The brains of people suffering from Alzheimer's disease also show three metabolic perturbations, or disturbances: these are inflammation, glycotoxicity (pathological changes caused by elevated levels of glucose), as well as other toxicity states, and loss of trophic (nutritional) support.

The brain of a person who does not have Alzheimer's disease is in what is medically known as a **synaptoblastic** condition. A synapse is the site of transmission of electric nerve impulses between two nerve cells (neurons), or between a neuron and a gland or muscle cell. So, synaptoblasts are healthy cells which are growing more "branches" to communicate with more nerves. These communicating "wires" are being grown in order to communicate more effectively and make the brain function optimally.

In the brain of a person with Alzheimer's disease, the environment is the opposite (**synaptoplastic**), where synapses cannot regenerate. This occurs because of inflammation, insulin-resistance, infections, low hormone levels, poor nutrition, mould, and toxic exposure.

The ultimate aim of treating Alzheimer's is therefore to increase synaptoplastic activity, i.e., to elevate the production of healthy nerve cells and restore – as far as possible – the efficiency of neural transmission within the brain.

A Multi-Pronged Condition Requiring a Multi-Pronged Treatment

We have seen above what the disease causes inside the brain. However, there are many different factors which contribute to a person developing the condition. It is a plurality spectrum – i.e., one condition with many imbalances and many pathways. For that reason, it cannot be treated with a one-size-fits-all, single approach. Every patient has their own specific profile, medical and genetic history, lifestyle and circumstances, and the treatment they receive must match that specific profile.

The "36 Holes in The Roof": The Imbalances of Alzheimer's Disease

Dr Dale Bredesen, an internationally recognised expert in the mechanisms of neurodegenerative diseases, has conducted extensive research into cognitive decline and Alzheimer's disease.

In his book *The End of Alzheimer's: The First Program to Prevent and Reverse Cognitive Decline* (Avery), he lays out a programme called "The Bredesen Protocol", in which he uses the metaphor of the "36 holes in the roof". Each of these "holes" is a metabolic imbalance, caused (or exacerbated) by either genetic, hormonal, environmental, dietary or lifestyle factors. Some of them may involve secondary imbalances. Through addressing each patient's individual challenges, Bredesen has created a targeted, individualised programme which works to correct up to 60 imbalances. In doing so, he has revolutionised conventional medicine's approach to the condition, which has failed abysmally. For many decades, medical practitioners have sought a single, enormous payday through a pharmaceutical monotherapy. This is an entirely unrealistic and impracticable quest, since Alzheimer's disease – as explained above – is on a pluralistic spectrum and requires a multi-pronged, individualised intervention for each patient's particular circumstances.

Repairing the "36 holes in the roof" (and their secondary imbalances) is not possible with a single therapy or drug which is good for any and every patient. Individuals with Alzheimer's disease are on different places on the spectrum and have developed the condition with varying degrees of severity, over different periods.

In an ideal world, a "silver bullet" Alzheimer's drug would be able to: reduce amyloid precursor protein (PP) cleavages (cell divisions) b and g, reduce caspase (protein enzymes which play a key role in cell death) cleavages 6 and 3, increase cleavage a, prevent oligomerisation (a chemical molecular process), increase neprilysin (a destructive enzyme), increase IDE (a binary chemical compound), increase microglial (tissue cells) clearance of Aβ (amino acids which are the main component of amyloid plaques found in the brains of people with Alzheimer's disease), increase autophagy (the body's way of cleaning out damaged cells), increase BDNF (a protein encoded in the BDNF gene), increase nerve growth factor, increase netrin-1 (a protein encoded in the NTN1 gene), increase ADNP (a gene which provides instructions for making a protein that helps control the activity of other genes), reduce homocysteine (an amino acid, high levels of which are linked to heart disease), increase PP2A (protein phosphatase 2, an enzyme encoded by the PPP2CA gene), reduce phospho-tau (an enzyme to which phosphate has been added), increase the phagocytosis index (a measure of counting the number of bacteria ingested), increase insulin sensitivity, improve the transport of axoplasm (a thick solution found within nerve cells), enhance mitochondrial function (i.e., regulate activity and biochemical reactions within cells) and biogenesis (the production of new living organisms), reduce oxidative damage, optimise the production of ROS (biochemical reactions), enhance cholinergic neurotransmission (functioning of nerve cells in which acetylcholine acts as a neurotransmitter), increase synaptoblastic signalling (communication between healthy cells), reduce synaptoclastic signalling (communication between unhealthy cells), increase long-term potentiation (persistent strengthening of healthy cells), optimise the hormones estradiol, progesterone, the E2:P ratio, optimise free T3 and T4 (tests of thyroid activity), optimise thyroid-stimulating activity, optimise the hormones pregnenolone, testosterone, cortisol, DHEA and insulin, reduce inflammation, increase resolvins (mediators that help control inflammation), enhance detoxification, improve vascularisation (the process in which body tissues develops capillaries), increase cAMP (cyclic adenosine monophosphate) – an important "messenger" in many biological processes, increase glutathione (an antioxidative substance produced by the liver), provide synaptic (healthy cell) components, optimise all metals, increase GABA (gamma aminobutyric acid, a naturally occurring amino acid which works as a neurotransmitter in the brain), increase vitamin D signalling, increase SirT1 (an enzyme in cell nuclei that contributes to cellular regeneration), reduce NFkB (a protein complex which causes inflammation), increase the length of telomeres (nucleotide sequences which protect the ends of chromosomes from deterioration or from fusion with neighbouring chromosomes), reduce glial scarring (scarring of non-neuronal cells in the brain and spine), enhance repair, etc.

We are sure that by now, you – the reader – feel understandably overwhelmed and alarmed. To anyone but a doctor or scientist, the above is a mind-boggling, tongue-twisting – and intimidating – list of boxes to tick. That is one of the reasons this book has been written – to demystify the condition of Alzheimer's disease (which, in truth, is considerably simpler than the above list suggests).

THE GOOD NEWS

While there is no denying that Alzheimer's is a terminal illness, it is equally true that that need not be the case. Although there is no "perfect Alzheimer's drug" capable of treating and correcting all of these itemised imbalances, the good news is that we do not need to wait for one. Bredesen found that the more "holes" in the roof we plug, the more likely we are to reverse cognitive decline.

What is more, there is a threshold effect: once a sufficient number of "holes" (critical point) is reached, reversal of the condition will **continue**, potentially achieving a significant improvement in functionality and memory of the patient.

Which of the 36 "holes" we plug depends on the variables presented by each patient's case. What is recommended for one patient may not be suitable for another, depending on age, medical history, circumstances, and other factors.

The symptoms of Alzheimer's disease worsen over time, although the rate at which the disease progresses varies considerably. The reality is that Alzheimer's disease is both largely preventable and treatable, using the **functional integrative medicine model.** This is a model which addresses the genetic, physiological, environmental, dietary, and psychological profile of each patient and is tailored to suit them, with the result that patients can live as long as 20 years, depending on a range of factors. It must be remembered that the disease is the result of a slow accumulation of neural changes, over years. This is referred to as pre-clinical Alzheimer's disease.

CAUSES OF ALZHEIMER'S DISEASE

The rate of cognitive decline is significantly linked to the kind of lifestyles we lead – including our diets, levels of activity, sleeping habits, stress levels and, particularly, our exposure to or consumption of **toxins.** Exposure to toxins such as alcohol, nicotine, chemicals found in drugs (both illicit and prescribed) and certain metals, as well as obesity, lack of exercise, insufficient sleep, stress, previous trauma affecting the brain and illnesses such as diabetes all aggravate the rate at which our memory retention is reduced. The factors of education (i.e., how informed we are of maintaining wellness) and economy (what is or is not accessible to us, given our financial status) are obviously important considerations. Our genetic profiles also play a significant role in predisposing us to the disease.

Let us look more closely at what these factors are and how they impact the human brain:

Nicotine

Apart from its carcinogenic effects on the body, particularly the lungs, nicotine decreases the blood flow to the brain, causing mental alertness to decline. It also upsets the balance between acetylcholine (the chemical released by nerve cells to send "messages" to other cells), leading to a lack of mental alertness. Since nicotine is among the most addictive of all drugs, legal and freely available in most parts of the world, it is one of the prime toxins contributing to the onset of Alzheimer's disease.

Alcohol

Like nicotine, alcohol is a drug which is not only easily available, but is socially endorsed and, indeed, accepted as an intrinsic accompaniment to meals, partying and business culture. However, alcohol negatively affects emotion and the processing of sensory information. It alters the activity of the hippocampus (a part of the brain situated in the temporal lobe which controls learning and memory) and disrupts the body's balance of serotonin, acetylcholine, and endorphins, causing depression and mood swings. Excessive alcohol abuse can damage the pancreas – the organ which converts the food we eat into fuel for the body's cells and whose endocrine function regulates its levels of blood sugar and production of insulin. Once this function is disrupted, diabetes can ensue – which, in turn, can trigger Alzheimer's disease.

Alcohol can cause depression, warp, and distort the ability to reason and impede sexual functioning. What is more, unsupervised, or abrupt withdrawal from regular, excessive alcohol consumption can cause delirium tremens, a traumatic neural event in which the brain – deprived of the drug on which it has come to depend – contracts like a sponge being squeezed dry. This can be fatal or cause lasting damage to the brain.

Adiposity (Excess Weight)

Adiposity is also a risk factor for Alzheimer's disease, particularly in middle age. In 2003, a study published in the *New England Journal of Medicine* showed that people who did ballroom dancing twice a week were less likely to develop dementia, while another study showed that for every extra mile walked per week, there was a 13% less chance of cognitive decline. Mid-life adiposity has been noted as a marker for Parkinson's disease in later life and body fat can act as a reservoir for neurotoxins that damage dopamine-producing neurons in the substantia nigra (the midbrain).

Poor Nutrition

Although the trend over the past decade towards healthy eating has been encouraging, populations in most Western countries, in particular, still consume regular – and large – amounts of convenience foods which are high in carbohydrates, fat and sugar, with little nutritional value. Fast-food meals typically contain highly processed (if any) vegetables or fruit, very little protein, and minimal vitamins, as well as certain toxins. Our modern, fast-paced lifestyles and the pressure of fitting job, home and social commitments into a typical working day leave little time for preparing wholesome meals, so we rely heavily on unhealthy snacks, or go for long periods without eating at all, only to over-compensate later by eating too much, too quickly. In South Africa, the majority of citizens are either unable to afford nutritious foods, or stick to traditional meals which consist almost entirely of starch and animal fats. A vitamin B deficiency (hyperhomocysteinaemia) can promote dementia by placing oxidative stress on the body, thickening the capillary walls of the blood vessels in the brain (thus causing them to leak protein and slow the flow of blood), shrinkage, fragmentation, and the eventual death of cells, as well as increasing amyloid toxicity.

Unhealthy eating is a significant contributing factor to cognitive decline. Ideally, a balanced, nutritious diet should include plenty of green and yellow vegetables (especially cooked kale and spinach), fruit (apples, blueberries, raspberries, blackberries, strawberries, cranberries, cherries, grapes, prunes, raisins), lean protein (fish, poultry, white meat, legumes, soya, cottage cheese), calcium (low-fat or skim milk), minimal carbohydrates (preferably unrefined starches such as wholemeal bread and brown rice), nuts (walnuts, almonds and pine nuts) and regular "good" fats (olive oil, seeds (pumpkin seeds, sunflower seeds, hemp seeds, flax seeds, sesame seeds, pistachio seeds), flax, Omega-3, Omega-7, Omega-9 and medium-chain triglyceride (MCT) oils – found in coconut and palm kernel).

Foods which are rich in phosphatidylserine (a phospholipid) are excellent for increasing neurotransmitters in the brain and therefore helping to maintain memory, attention, and concentration beyond early middle age. These foods include fish, rice, soy, and green leafy vegetables such as spinach.

Refined sugar should be avoided, even though it has become a ubiquitous ingredient in so many modern

lifestyles. A study has found that the average American consumes 63-72kg of sugar a year, while the average South African consumes 12-24 teaspoons of sugar a day. Four to eight
of these teaspoons are found in sweetened beverages such
as coffee, tea, and mineral drinks. Sugar depletes the body
of B vitamins and calcium and promotes inflammation by
increasing the production of free radicals (oxygen-contain-
ing molecules with an uneven number of electrons, which
can cause large chain reactions in the body by reacting easily
with other molecules). These reactions are called oxidation.
It is essential to achieve a balance between free radicals and
antioxidants for proper physiological functioning, because
if free radicals overwhelm the body's ability to regulate them,
oxidative stress results, adversely impacting lipids, proteins
and DNA and causing a number of diseases, including
cancer.

It is also important to avoid "bad" oils (processed or
hydrogenated oils) and fatty meats, as these cause plaque
to build up in narrow blood vessels, decreasing the blood
flow to the brain and increasing the risk of heart disease
and stroke. Saturated fatty acids interfere with glucose, the
main fuelling source in the brain.

Lack of Exercise

Lack of exercise is a global problem, particularly in Western countries, where work pressures, family and social

commitments invariably make physical activity a "nice-to-do", rather than a regular habit. In South Africa, this is compounded by high crime rates, with many people unwilling to walk, jog or cycle in open or unguarded spaces. The preoccupation with digital technology – including gaming, social media platforms and the Internet – has also become a recreational priority, especially among youngsters. Yet regular exercise is essential for the health of the entire body, including the brain. Lack of physical (and mental) exercise causes loss of physical function. Exercise increases the blood flow and the release of mood-regulating neurotransmitters, stimulates new neuron growth, and strengthens neural connections. People who play sport, go to gym, or take up some form of regular physical activity enjoy better metabolic functioning, improved cardiac and psychological health and better weight control. This helps prevent mid-life adiposity.

Sleep Deprivation

Sleep is crucial to brain health. Sleep deprivation impedes emotional and psychological well-being, as well as impacting the brain by decreasing memory. The body's immune system, detoxification and lymphatic system all operate better during sleep.

Factors causing sleep deprivation include illness, stimulants such as drugs, coffee (caffeine) and aspartame (an artificial, non-saccharide sweetener, which is neurotoxic). These also deprive the body of B vitamins and can cause tremors and anxiety.

There are four distinct stages to sleep: Stage 1 is light sleep (approximately 2-5% of total sleep time). Stage 2 is low-voltage, mixed-frequency electric activity in the brain (approximately 45-55% of sleep time); Stage 3 is slow-wave sleep (25-50% high-voltage waves of electrical activity in the brain); and Stage 4 is more than 50% of high-voltage waves of electrical activity in the brain). Rapid-eye-movement (REM) sleep represents 20-25% of total sleep time and in this state, electrical brain activity is desynchronised, while the rest of the body shows muscle inhibition. There are also intermittent muscular twitches and eye movements.

Poor sleep at night leads to changes in mood and emotions, as well as behaviour. Aggressiveness, weak memory, confusion, and an inability to think clearly are typical, while there is a clear decline in academic and social performance.

As we get older, the quality of sleep invariably worsens. There is decreased REM sleep, decreased slow-wave sleep and increased stage shifts.

Sleep disorders include restless leg syndrome (an inability to fall or remain asleep), triggering a need to get up and walk around and then, the next day, sleepiness. This syndrome is common in people with neuropathies and myelopathies (spinal cord injuries), pregnancy, anaemia, renal failure, a deficiency in magnesium, B12 and folate, habitual intake of caffeine (especially at night), medications such as tricycylic or selective serotonin re-uptake inhibiting anti-depressants, obesity, an underactive thyroid gland, and low dopamine levels.

During menopause, sleep is often disturbed by "hot flushes" and night sweats, mood swings, anxiety attacks, depression, and low progesterone levels.

Mould

A variety of moulds are found in water-damaged buildings and other damp environments. The foreign antigens they produce remain in the body, causing the immune system to continually fight back. This causes inflammation in the body and results in chronic illness and massive hormonal disruption.

The symptoms of mould infections include fatigue, aphasia (difficulty finding words), memory loss, weakness, achiness, headaches, sensitivity to light, inability to concentrate, cramps and stiffness, tingling of the skin, sinus congestion, shortness of breath, coughing, increased thirst, confusion, appetite swings, frequent and/or urgent urination, irregular body temperature, blurry vision, excessive sweating (or night sweats), mood swings, diarrhoea, abdominal tenderness, a metallic taste in the mouth and vertigo (dizziness).

Other Toxins

These include:

- *cyanobacteria*, which come from freshwater blue-green algae and can cause neural, liver, skin and gastro-intestinal complications

- the *Ciguatera* toxin, which moves up the ocean food chain into feeder fish and then into larger predatory species such as red snappers, groupers, and barracuda

- *ionophoric* toxins, which are miniscule and can move easily in and out of cells, but are difficult to detect in the blood. In people who are genetically susceptible to toxins, the body is unable to eliminate them, so they can lead to chronic stimulation of the immune system. This results in dysfunction in the cells and an inability to process glucose

- it also leads to gliotoxicity, which is produced by fungus and suppresses the immune system by inhibiting the production of white blood cells in the body and interfering with other metabolic processes.

HORMONAL DECLINE AND IMBALANCE

All the body's hormones work in unison. Some may work in one direction, others in another direction, but they always work towards homeostasis (hormonal balance), without which there can be no true or sustainable state of health.

However, ageing is a process in which there is natural hormonal decline, particularly after mid-life. The hormones which are crucial to maintaining memory and cognitive ability are:

Estrogen

Estrogen enhances verbal memory (the ability to remember words) and the ability to learn and recall new material. It also increases nerve growth, increases the production of acetylcholine (the chief neural transmitter in the nervous system), stimulates an increase in dopamine receptors (which modulate spatial working memory), helps prevent the deposit of beta-amyloids (the main components of plaque found in the brains of people with Alzheimer's disease), increases blood flow and helps protect the hippocampus (the part of the brain which plays a major part in learning and memory).

Thyroid Hormone

Thyroid hormones, produced by the thyroid gland, help maintain memory, as well as overall metabolic functioning. Low thyroid levels directly cause low pregnenolone levels. Thyroid function naturally decreases with age (typically from 45-50), but can also be impaired by deficiencies of vitamin D, ferritin (a blood protein which contains iron), cortisol, iodine, and tyrosine (particularly in vegans, vegetarians, and bodybuilders).

DHEA (Dehydroepiandrosterone)

DHEA is a hormone produced by the adrenal glands which helps prevent depression and other psychological conditions, obesity, and diseases such as lupus, osteoporosis, vaginal atrophy, and erectile dysfunction. Low DHEA levels caused by ageing and stress can reduce the memory and lead to cognitive decline. Patients with Alzheimer's disease have been found to have levels of DHEA which are 48% lower than in non-patients. Deficiencies can also cause impaired immune responses, leading to chronic infections and allergies, arthritis and sclerosis, stress, depression, cognitive decline, heart disease, muscle loss and homocysteine (an amino acid found in meat which, in high levels, can lead to heart disease, vitamin deficiencies and renal disease).

Pregnenolone

This is the hormone controlling nerve transmission and memory in the body. It regulates the balance between excitation and inhibition in the nervous system (i.e., the response to sensory, tactile, and emotional stimuli), increases resistance to stress, improves mental and physical energy, directly influences the release of acetylcholine, reduces pain and inflammation, and blocks the formation of harmful acid-forming compounds. It is necessary for the formation of DHEA, estrogen, progesterone and testosterone, all of which decline with age. By the age of 75, most people have 65% less pregnenolone than they did at age 36.

Progesterone

Progesterone (known mainly as a female sex hormone) is made up of protein and fatty substances. It is produced in the brain, spinal cord and peripheral nervous system and promotes the formation of myelin sheaths, the insulating layers that form around nerve fibres, allowing electrical impulses to be transmitted quickly and efficiently along the nerve cells to the brain. This, in turn, enables proper motor and cognitive functioning.

Melatonin

Melatonin is a hormone which is an antioxidant and neurotransmitter. It assists with sleep, helps prevent cardiovascular disorders and boosts the immunity. Patients with Alzheimer's disease have lower levels of melatonin.

Cortisol

Both high and low levels of cortisol – which is produced by stress – affect memory. Since stress is an inevitable part of life, the solution is not to try to eliminate it, but to learn healthy ways of coping with it.

A lack of cortisol (adrenocortical insufficiency) can be treated with hydrocortisone, which is the name for the hormone cortisol in medicated form. It must be administered carefully, in doses which do not induce thyroid absorption issues, but which effectively address acute stress, low blood sugar levels or impending illnesses such as rheumatoid arthritis, dermatitis, asthma and chronic obstructive pulmonary disorder.

Growth Hormone (GH)

Levels of the growth hormone peak during puberty and begin to decrease at the age of 21. By the age of 60, during a period of 24 hours, most adults secrete hormones at the same rate at which someone with lesions in their pituitary gland would be secreting them. The loss of GH causes muscular weakness, weak bones, loss of skeletal muscle mass, increased total and abdominal fat, glucose intolerance, high cholesterol levels, fragility of the skin and blood vessels, decreased immune function and overall decreased quality of life.

Testosterone

There are special cells in the testes that produce testosterone, while a small amount is produced in the adrenal glands.

The entire body has testosterone receptors, including the brain, and the hormone is carried in the blood bound to carrier molecules. During andropause (male menopause), the loss of testosterone is typically very slow and subtle, with symptoms accepted as inevitable results of ageing. These include loss of libido, erectile and orgasmic dysfunction, a reduced amount of ejaculatory fluid and reduced intensity of orgasm. Non-sexual symptoms include increased fatigue, depression, irritability, night sweats and difficulty sleeping. Muscle strength and mass are lost, fat accumulates (particularly in the abdomen), bone density is lost, anaemia may develop, body and scalp hair are reduced and there is a heightened risk of cardiovascular disease.

All these hormones are hugely beneficial for trophic (activity-stimulating) support of the brain.

Deprived of that trophic support, the body goes into adrenal stress and burnout (hypoadrenia), where a person experiences fatigue, impaired memory, insomnia or disturbed sleep, depression, sugar craving, low blood sugar and low blood pressure, weaker immunity to infections and diseases, irritability, digestive problems, muscle and joint pain and glandular imbalances which can affect the thyroid and cause pre-menstrual and menopausal syndrome, as well as impacting fertility.

Besides the nutrient supports listed above, adrenocortical insufficiency can be treated with hydrocortisone, which is the name for the cortisol hormone in medicated form. It must be administered carefully, in doses which do not induce thyroid absorption issues, but which effectively address acute stress, low blood sugar levels or impending illnesses such as rheumatoid arthritis, dermatitis, asthma and chronic obstructive pulmonary disorder.

What causes adrenal stress? Long periods of stress, nutritional deficiency, untreated or undiagnosed hypothyroidism, exposure to toxic metals and halogens (e.g., fluoride, chlorine, and bromine).

Again, the above lengthy list of hormonal processes is not intended to intimidate the reader, but simply to explain their complexity. The interplay of their essential activities is intricate and balancing them is crucial, as a single imbalance can affect the entire metabolism. The best metaphor would be a philharmonic orchestra: a piece of classical music is played in which the listener is often aware of only the most prominently audible or visible instruments (the strings and horns). Yet if even one comparatively unnoticed instrument (e.g., a triangle, a double bass, a wind chime, or a glockenspiel) is late in playing a note, or is missing from the orchestra, the listener would immediately hear that something was wrong or missing.

Neurotransmitters

Serotonin

Serotonin (5-hydroxytryptamine) is a hormone with complex and multi-faceted functions, including modulating mood, cognition, learning, memory, and physiological processes such as vasoconstriction and vomiting. Lack of serotonin results in sleep disorders, depression, fatigue or lethargy, obsessive-compulsive behaviours, sugar or carbohydrate cravings, irritable bowel syndrome, premenstrual tension, and pain. The hormone can be replenished by taking magnesium glycinate, SAMe and Super Mega B supplements.

Dopamine

This neurotransmitter triggers motivation, enthusiasm, energy, self-confidence, pleasure, self-discipline, and sexual function. Lack of it results in fatigue, addictions, depression, attention disorders, hyperactivity, and obesity. A deficiency of it can be corrected by taking tyrosine, ginkgo biloba, SAMe and Stress Damage Control supplements.

Noradrenaline

Noradrenaline controls attention, vigilance, focus, sweating, blood pressure and the "fight-or-flight" response in threatening situations. A lack of it results in an inability to cope with stress, low blood pressure and abnormal temperature regulation, causing a loss of sweating. It can be found in the supplements L-phenylalanine, SAMe and Super Mega B.

Acetylcholine

This neurotransmitter helps control memory, learning, information processing and language. Lack of it results in poor memory (including in elderly individuals), agitation, loss of creativity and learning disorders. Acetylcholine can be found in the supplements Krill Oil, DMAE, acetyl-L-carnitine, phosphatidyl serine and Gingko biloba.

Gamma-Aminobutyric Acid (Gaba)

This neurotransmitter helps to regulate calmness and contentedness and control anxiety. Lack of it can result in tremors, anxiety, sleep disturbances, tension, cardiac arrhythmias, phobias, restlessness, and high blood pressure. A deficiency of GABA can be corrected by taking theanine, inositol, magnesium glycinate, taurine, N-acetylcysteine, and melatonin.

Amino Acids

Amino acids are not hormones, but neurotransmitters which are essential for healthy functioning of the sex hormones and thyroid.

Stress

Stress is an unavoidable, but manageable part of modern life, particularly in urban settings. Apart from affecting the capacity to function by distorting one's perceptions of, and response to, situations, it can disrupt sleep and rewire the emotional circuits of the brain, destroying nerve connections (neurons).

In a situation of anxiety or fear, the adrenal glands release cortisol – the primary stress hormone – as part of the fight-flight-or-freeze reaction. Cortisol, in turn, causes heightened levels of breathing, an increased heart rate and the release of sugars (glucose) into the bloodstream. However, high levels of cortisol – caused by stress – can result in the atrophy and death of neurons by causing the brain to produce an inflammatory marker called Interleukin-6 (IL-6), which is increased in the brains of patients with cognitive decline.

While nobody can avoid situations of stress, a lot can be done to control it by learning to recognise what triggers it and ways of relaxing in such situations, such as deep breathing. It is also essential to give one's body and brain a fighting chance of dealing with stress by getting adequate sleep, doing regular exercise, having regular periods of leisure, and following a nutritious, balanced diet.

Food Allergies

When the body has an allergic reaction to something, the immune system tries to fight it. This causes an inflammatory response. If the source of the allergy is not handled, but merely suppressed, the immune system will continue fighting, causing chronic inflammation which can lead to serious illnesses such as inflammatory bowel disease, rheumatoid arthritis, eczema, lupus, multiple sclerosis, asthma, coronary artery disease, diabetes – and also dementia, which is the breakdown of cognitive functioning in the brain.

The most common allergens affecting the brain are sugar, tomatoes, wheat, coffee, dairy products, peanuts, beef, soy nuts, potatoes, corn, shellfish, yeast, and eggs. Nutrients used to treat these allergies are commonly vitamin c, anti-inflammatories such as bromelain and MSM (methylsulfonylmethane), methionine and chamomile (which reduce histamine levels), glutamine (which increases GABA (gamma aminobutyric acid, a naturally occurring amino acid that works as a neurotransmitter in the brain) and goldenseal (*Hydrastis canadensis*), a plant native to eastern North America whose roots and leaves are commonly used by native Americans to treat allergies and inflammations.

Drugs

There is a common misconception that over-the-counter drugs, which are legal, inexpensive, and easy to obtain, are harmless. While they indeed have a necessary and useful role to play in offering the public relief for a very wide range of complaints, the fact remains that they are chemical compounds which impact the body.

Used excessively or injudiciously, *recreational, prescribed, and over-the-counter drugs* can *all* cause damage to neural functioning. These include analgesics (pain-relievers), anti-arrhythmic drugs (for cardiac disorders), antibiotics, anti-convulsants, anti-depressants, antihistamines and decongestants, antihypertensive drugs (used to control high blood pressure), levodopa (commonly used to treat Parkinson's disease), steroids, muscle relaxants, sedatives, and statin medications.

Anti-cholinergic drugs (e.g. those used to treat urinary incontinence), anti-spasmodics (to treat intestinal cramps or bladder symptoms), cold and cough medications, antacids (for heartburn and stomach pain), anti-dysrhythmics (used to treat cardiac arrhythmias), anti-emetics (to prevent vomiting), anti-psychotics (to treat a range of psychiatric illnesses) and anti-Parkinsonian drugs (to treat tremors and other effects of Parkinson's disease, as well as related disorders) can also all impact memory and cognitive function in later life, especially if they are used over long periods. This applies equally to eye, ear, and nose drops, as well as herbal preparations.

Always know what you or your family are taking and why. Ask about the long-term effects of the drug or medication, as well as its side-effects.

The harmful effects of the four main categories of *illicit drugs* (stimulants such as cocaine, depressants such as barbiturates, opioids such as heroin and hallucinogens such as LSD and cannabis) are exacerbated by a wide and continually mutating category of recreational street drugs (tik, nyaope, Ecstasy, crack cocaine, crystal meth, etc) – which are generally cheap and extremely dangerous.

Vaccines

Vaccines are a contentious subject when it comes to brain inflammation. While they have saved millions of lives by preventing killer diseases (including, hopefully, the current Covid-19 virus), the fact remains that most vaccines contain an antigen, combined with chemicals that stimulate the immune system, called adjuvants. A good example is the hepatitis vaccine, which contains a genetically engineered version of the virus, along with aluminium salts as adjuvants. The inflammation caused by the adjuvants is specific for that antigen (just as a pharmaceutical product affects only its target and leaves the rest of the body alone), so this targeted inflammation offers protection from that particular threat (in this case, hepatitis). This reasoning has been used for the past 200 years in the way vaccines are made.

However, modern research has found that the immune system is considerably more complex than was first understood. Specifically, three scientific discoveries – of the microbiome, exosomes and the role of psychology, or belief in medical outcomes – have altered the way we view vaccines.

The *microbiome* is the collection of trillions of microbes such as bacteria, fungi and viruses which live in and on us. These are by no means all bad: they perform functions vital to our well-being and survival, including digestion, nutrient assimilation, and hormone production. What is more, the fast evolution of microbes helps us adapt to changing threats – for example, gut bacteria help us detoxify cleaning chemicals. For this reason, vaccines need to be designed to work with our highly complex human microbe ecosystem.

Exosomes are tiny vesicles that our cells secrete to communicate across long distances in the body. They contain proteins, RNA, DNA, and other signalling molecules that influence genetic expression. Exosomes are being intensely researched in the context of brain health, especially neurodegenerative and psychiatric diseases. Although this research is still in its early stages, it is known that toxins like mercury and aluminium (which are contained in vaccines) trigger the release of exosomes that send "danger signals". This suggests that vaccines enter the exosome network in disruptive ways which we simply do not understand.

The role of *psychology and beliefs* has long been underestimated in medicine, especially in the area of immunity to diseases. The strong connection between the mind and the body (for example, the way a patient who is unaware that they are taking a placebo, rather than a genuine medication, often still recovers because they believe they will) is undeniable. The placebo effect has been remarkable in mending broken bones, relieving depression and insomnia, and extending the life of cancer patients. Vaccines offer no opportunity for us to trust our bodies to ward off disease – a fear-based approach which undermines the very beliefs that enable true health.

The ingredients of vaccines include preservatives, stabilisers, sugars (which negatively impact muscle cells), gelatin and egg proteins (both allergens), residual cell culture materials, residual inactivating ingredients, formaldehyde (a known carcinogen), residual antibiotics (which are designed to kill cells), detergents, monosodium glutamate and foreign proteins which can activate a variety of unpredictable immune responses. Furthermore, several vaccines contain "weakened' versions of the viruses they are designed to ward off. These can activate latent viruses in the body which would otherwise be harmless. This chain reaction has been linked to schizophrenia and bipolar disorder.

Antibiotics in vaccines can kill beneficial bacteria in the microbiome, which controls 70-80% of immune responses.

Aluminium is contained in at least 18 vaccines, including those advised (or enforced) for infants. Aluminium can remain in the body for years and has been strongly linked to chronic fatigue and cognitive decline, among other disorders. It is also a risk factor for autoimmunity, long-term brain inflammation and associated neurological complications.

Multi-dose vials of the flu vaccine contain thimerosal, a mercury-based preservative. Mercury is a known neurotoxin. Furthermore, the flu vaccine is notoriously ineffective, with the current estimate of 48% effectiveness against only a few strains of many. One study showed that the flu vaccine actually hampered the body's immunity, while another showed that the vaccine made recipients more susceptible to contracting an even worse version of the virus, H1N1 (swine flu).

Having noted all of this, we must add that a blanket approach against all vaccinations is equally dangerous. The solution is a middle path through both extremes, combining the best of medical science with temperance. Adjustments could be made in the *timing* of vaccines – for example, vaccinating a child at the age of three or four months, rather than at birth (unless, of course, the mother is ill herself, which creates a totally different situation), or administering a vaccine against a single specific disease at spaced-out times, rather than a triple vaccine at one time against diphtheria, tetanus, and pertussis, or against rubella, measles, and mumps.

Addiction and the "Hijacked Brain"

There is a wide range of substances and behaviours to which people become addicted, from alcohol, nicotine, recreational drugs, sugar and other foodstuffs to coffee, gambling, sexual promiscuity, cell phones, social media platforms, shopping and more.

Addiction is the fastest-growing pandemic in the world. It is also the most democratic one, since it affects people of all ages, cultures, ethnicities, educational backgrounds, professions, income brackets and faiths. It impacts not only users, but their families, their communities, and their employers. Substance use (including alcohol, illicit drugs, and nicotine) was responsible for 11,8 million deaths globally in 2017 (which equates to one in five deaths), yet the crisis of addiction remains a low priority in many of the most affected countries. It is habitually outsourced to either the state, the criminal justice system, or the churches to deal with, or it is simply ignored as an "aberration" or a self-inflicted condition whose consequences addicts "deserve" because "they chose to do it".

There are seven pervasive **myths** responsible for this attitude:

- "Compulsive use of an addictive substance or behaviour is a sign or weakness or poor moral character."

- "Chronic addiction is a disease that can be treated with prescription drugs."

- *"Drugs and alcohol are the cause of substance abuse."* (The converse is true: they are the *result*, or end-stage, of an addicted mindset, not the cause of it.)

- "Avoiding relapse will always be a constant struggle for recovering substance abusers."

- "Substance abuse is genetic." ("It runs in my family, so I can't help it.")

- *"Shame, guilt and punishment are the most effective tools for getting addicts to stop."* (In fact, they do not cure addiction – they *cause* it, since a distressed or anxious addict will immediately seek emotional relief or escape in their substance or behaviour of choice.)

- *"Addiction is a choice, not an illness."* (In fact, it is an illness **of** choice. An addicted mind is unable to make choices, because it is driven by compulsion, rather than reason.)

- *"They could stop if they really wanted to."* (Of course, they "really want to". Addiction is not fun. No addict enjoys the downward spiral, humiliation, misery, and stigma in which they are trapped: nor does anyone "plan" to become an addict.) However, addiction is a disease which operates from the primal area of the brain that is concerned with sheer survival, not with logic.

"Addiction hijacks the pleasure pathways of the brain. It looks for things/thought/emotions to get high over and if all is calm, it will create chaos. Addiction is an impulsive and irrational disease. It does not exist in the frontal lobe of the brain, where reasoning and logic are. Addiction lives in the mid-brain, the amygdala, where fight-flight are found. This part of the brain trumps reasoning, every time." – Lorelie Razzano, www.jaggedlittleedges.com

The Origins of Addiction

Addiction progresses through four distinct stages. The first is experimental, when the user tries a substance, enjoys it, and occasionally indulges in it. ("I *like* to use it.") The second is the stage where the user feels a more frequent desire for it and begins to actively seek it out ("I *want* to use it.") The third stage is where the user relies on the drug to perform daily functions, such as their job or social obligations ("I *need* to use it"). The final stage is where the user is unable to function at all without it and is totally obsessed with obtaining it ("I *have* to use it"). By this final stage, an addict has no alternative but to satisfy their craving, even if this means stealing, lying, assaulting, or begging for it. An addict craving a fix is in the same mental state as a ravenous concentration camp inmate so desperate for food that they will resort to cannibalism, coprophagia, stealing, lying, begging, assault or murder to obtain it.

Some people are able to maintain a state of functional addiction for extended periods – i.e., they can continue working, socialising, and coping with their daily demands, balancing these with their addiction. However, sooner or later, the spiral descends

The Reward Deficiency Syndrome

In the addicted or "hijacked" brain, the pleasure centre releases the neurotransmitter dopamine, which activates the reward centre in the brain, as well as serotonin (the "feel-good" hormone). The brain remembers these as "pleasure signals" and retains them in the same areas associated with normal reward processing. The end result is the same: there is a rise of blood glucose and dopamine, to which the brain becomes addicted. Once the addictive substance is unavailable to the user, the lack of dopamine in the reward centre of the brain causes a feeling of being unwell, threatened, or unhappy, and the addict begins to experience craving.

Causes of The Reward Deficiency Syndrome

- Genetic factors. Research has found that the endorphins released in response to drinking bind to a specific opioid receptor, the Mu receptor. Some individuals are more susceptible to alcohol abuse because they have different levels of endorphins. Beta-endorphins – which are a type of "morphine", or "endogenous analgesic" released by the brain in response to certain situations, such as numbing extreme pain (e.g., someone who has survived a shark attack, but only begins to feel their injuries after the event) – are a useful biological marker to identify these individuals. A lack of endorphins is hereditary.

- Past traumas (either emotional or physical) and severe, protracted stress.

- Environmental factors, such as a lack of nutrients, long-term sleep deprivation or prenatal conditions.

- Peer pressure, insecurity, or depression.

- Heavy use of addictive substances (including food, prescription medications, recreational drugs, or alcohol). Psychoactive substances fit into the same neurotransmitter receptors as natural brain chemicals, but work faster and better.

- For a person with reward deficiency syndrome, addictive substances, or behaviours (temporarily) provide what they cannot find elsewhere: relief, enhanced performance, self-confidence, calm, stimulation, a sense of belonging to a peer group, etc.

- Others are triggered by *abstinence* from a substance (withdrawal, craving and seeking behaviours).

Glutamate in Addiction

Until recently, addiction research in neuroscience focused on mechanisms involving only dopamine and endogenous opioids. Now researchers have realised that glutamate also plays a central role in the processes underlying the development and maintenance of addiction. These processes include reinforcement, sensitisation, habit-learning, context conditioning, craving and relapse. It has been well documented that in many cases, addicts who successfully withdraw from one drug or behaviour simply replace it with another.

Conventional Treatments in Addiction

Counselling and education: Psychotherapy or behavioural-cognitive modification, recovery wellness coaching, offered by rehabilitation centres, hospitals, medical practitioners, and psychologists.

Support groups: Examples are Alcoholics Anonymous, Narcotics Anonymous and faith- or community-based groups for addicts and their co-dependants.

Prescription medications: These include naltrexone, anti-depressants, mood stabilisers, sleep aids and tranquillisers. In several countries, addicts are able to register under recovery programmes where they are given free methadone (a synthetic opioid used for opioid maintenance therapy and for chronic pain management, sold under the brand names Dolophine and Methadose, among other). The methadone is given in decreasing dosages for a limited period to help the addict cope with the extreme physical and mental pain and cravings associated with withdrawal from heroin. Methadone changes the way the brain and nervous system respond to pain, though its effects are slower and weaker than those of other analgesics like morphine. It also blocks the "high" the addict experiences from drugs like codeine, heroin, hydrocodone, morphine, and oxycodone, but delivers a similar (if weaker) feeling. This is sometimes called "replacement therapy", but it is not a cure, as it addresses only the symptoms, rather than the causes of addiction. It is simply one measure used to detoxify addicts (who then frequently relapse and in due course need to return for a second, third or fourth course of methadone).

It should be noted that these traditional/conventional treatments have seldom included routine, science-based dietary and nutritional interventions for addiction.

Integrative Therapies for Addiction

Notable success in treatment has been achieved by combining therapies, thus addressing several aspects of the addict's recovery. Some examples of this are:

- Counselling + education + recovery wellness coaching + support groups such as Alcoholics Anonymous or Narcotics Anonymous.

- Six to 10 days of intravenous or oral nutrient therapy.

- Healthy eating + daily oral supplementation (nutrients for healing the brain and the liver, as well as for improving sleep).

- Stress/Cortisol therapy + exercise, meditation, and yoga.

- Fatty acid analysis.

- Weaning depression medication.

- Food sensitivity and coeliac disease evaluation and treatment.

The Untreated Brain

Someone who is in active addiction or who is still in denial about their problem usually finds it difficult to focus on or fully benefit from support groups, counselling, recovery wellness coaching or other forms of therapy. Deprived of their addictive substance or behaviour, they are generally angry, defensive, and ashamed, while also having to cope with the anger and anxiety of their family or co-dependants. This often results in the addict either dropping out of a treatment programme or simply "sticking it out" (to pacify their family or partner), while already planning their next "fix" as soon as the opportunity arises.

It is crucial to understand that an addict only contemplates asking for help when they are not actively craving – i.e., when they are not coping with the traumatic experience of withdrawal. Once they are craving their substance or behaviour, they are focused solely on finding a way to get it. Thus, the window of rationality is very small and becomes increasingly smaller as the addict requires more and more of their substance to maintain a sense of well-being.

Restoring and Regulating Normal Transmitter Balance

The neurotransmitters involved in addiction and relapse are dopamine, serotonin, noradrenaline, GABA, taurine, opioids, and glutathione. Neurotransmitters are literally made of nutrients – amino acids, vitamins, and minerals – and it is possible to formulate the ideal "brain food" to restore them and break the cycle of addiction.

Nutritional supplements are able to restore balance and create a state of high energy, increased focus, and well-being, without excessive withdrawal cravings, pain, or side-effects. The nutrients provide the brain cells with exactly what they need to operate optimally fairly quickly.

Dopamine and noradrenaline stimulate the brain and elevate the mood. Serotonin and GABA also elevate the mood, while calming anxiety and agitation. Acetylcholine enhances the memory and general cognitive ability.

While the addict is taking a course of nutritional supplements, it is also necessary to identify stimulants that could "trigger" them and limit their exposure to them (e.g., friends with whom they drank or used drugs, places where they did this, parties, etc). They should also follow a healthy, low-GI diet and get regular exercise. And, crucially, there should be complete abstinence from the addictive substance.

Should cravings become strong, 500mg of L-glutamine taken sublingually is quickly absorbed and delivers a "pick-up" similar to that of the craved stimulant. The dosage may be given several times a day, between meals. L-glutamine also reduces carbohydrate cravings by raising the brain blood glucose and reduces food allergies by repairing the lining of the gastro-intestinal tract, which is often inflamed in alcoholics.

Treating Alcoholism with Nutrients

- Niacin is the single most important – and most reliable – treatment for alcoholism.

- L-glutamine (2 000mg or 3 000mg) reduces the physiological craving for alcohol. It is naturally produced in the liver and kidneys – both organs which are damaged by alcohol abuse – so supplementation is vital. L-glutamine also reduces the craving for sugar.

- Lecithin (30-60ml daily) provides inositol and choline.

- Chromium (at least 200-400mcg daily) is highly effective in controlling blood sugar levels (which are low in many alcoholics).

- Vitamin C should be taken to saturation (i.e., 10 000-20 000mg per day or more). This chemically neutralises the toxic breakdown products of alcohol metabolism. Vitamin C also boosts the liver's ability to reverse the fatty build-up which is common in alcoholics. A dose of 1 000mg of vitamin C, taken every hour, will result in a single episode of diarrhoea. Thereafter, the same dosage should be given every four hours.

- Vitamin B complex containing each of the major B vitamins, especially B1.

- A high-potency multi-vitamin, multi-mineral supplement should also be given. It should contain magnesium (400mg) and the antioxidants carotene and d-alpha tocopherol.

- The "Sinclair method" – an evidence-based treatment for alcoholism developed by American physician John D Sinclair – is unique in that, unlike other therapies which require complete abstinence, it requires the patient to continue drinking alcohol at the beginning of the treatment, in combination with naltrexone. The naltrexone, which is taken one hour before the first drink of the day, prevents endorphins (the natural opiates in the brain) from being released when the alcohol is imbibed. There is therefore no "buzz" or rewarding, pleasurable feeling that drives an alcoholic to drink excessively. Continued over time, the brain learns not to associate alcohol with enjoyment or relief, resulting in reduced cravings.

- Acetyl-L-carnitine may also reduce the craving for alcohol by reducing the severity of withdrawal symptoms.

Treating Nicotine Addiction with Nutrients

- Nicotine decreases the blood flow to the brain. It also induces the brain cells to develop nicotinic receptors that respond to acetylcholine. However, as acetylcholine production continues rapidly, the balance between the neurotransmitters is upset.

- Daily doses of vitamin C (1 000mg), chromium, niacin (B3), calcium (about 500mg) and magnesium (about 500mg), 5-hydroxytryptophan (5HTP) (200mg) and St John's Wort (300mg of the "standardised extract" three times daily, after food, commencing one week before the date chosen for cessation of smoking and continuing for three to four months).

Treating Chocolate Addiction with Nutrients

- Chocolate – known as the "love drug" – contains phenylethylamine, a brain stimulant producing a feeling of pleasure.

- The nutrient used to address this is DL-phenylalanine (500-1 000mg twice or three times daily).

- Omega-3 in fish or flax oil should also be taken.

- A low-sugar diet should be followed.

Treating Benzodiazepine Addiction with Nutrients

- Benzodiazepines are tranquillising drugs (e.g., Valium, Xanax) which become addictive in as little as four weeks of regular use. While they deliver a sense of relaxation and calmness, there is generally grogginess and a "hung-over" feeling the next day. The withdrawal symptoms include insomnia, anxiety, irritability, sweating, blurred vision, depression, tremors, lack of mental focus and headaches. The recommended treatment here is:

- Theanine (300mg twice daily).

- Melatonin (1-6mg daily). (It is also useful in treating insomnia.)

- Valerian (5-100mg twice or three times daily).

- Glycine, corydalis, passionflower, and magnesium.

Treating Recreational Drug Addiction with Nutrients

- Ecstasy is often taken by youngsters at all-night concerts or parties since it dramatically boosts energy levels for up to 12 hours. If the user is continually active during that period (e.g., dancing), the result is often severe dehydration, which can be fatal. It depletes the body of serotonin by causing excessive amounts to be produced.

- Opiates (morphine, codeine, opium, etc). Opiates slow down the respiratory system, which slows down breathing. Nerve cells in the brain naturally produce opiates, which act as painkillers or endorphins, and also reduce histamine. A person using an opiate develops a tolerance to it and then requires more and more of it to produce the same effect. This prevents the nerve cells in the brain from producing natural opiates. Excessive use of these drugs can completely shut down the respiratory system, resulting in death.

- Cocaine and amphetamines block serotonin and noradrenaline. This prevents the uptake of dopamine.

- Supplements should include 5-HTP (100mg three times a day), tyrosine (up to 5 000mg daily) and S-adenosyl methionine (SAMe) (400-1 600mg daily).

- Tryptophan (4 000mg per day) may also be useful in facilitating the production of serotonin and reducing the pain and anxiety caused by withdrawal.

- Oxytocin has been found to help prevent the development of tolerance to opiates and alcohol.

- Carnosine may help prevent addiction to morphine, alcohol, sugary foods, and carbohydrates.

- Low progesterone levels are common among drug addicts and alcoholics. As many as 40% of middle-aged female addicts were shown to have this deficiency. When progesterone levels are restored, anxiety and insomnia in recovering addicts are reduced, which in turn subdues craving.

Treating Gambling and Drug Addiction with Nutrients

Medical studies have shown that N-acetylcysteine (NAC) reduces the compulsion in both gamblers and drug addicts to gamble or use. It does this by reducing their withdrawal symptoms and cravings (particularly those associated with cocaine and marijuana addiction). It is thought to have a role as an antioxidant and supports the liver, promotes detoxification, and chelates heavy metals. NAC has also been investigated as a treatment for nicotine addiction.

Maintaining Recovery with Nutrients

- Low levels of docosahaenoic acid (DHA) – a type of Omega-3 fat – may increase vulnerability to relapse after successful abstinence, particularly in cocaine addicts.

- There is evidence that polyunsaturated fatty acids – which influence the central serotonergic and dopaminergic systems, both involved in the brain's reward mechanism – could play a role in substance addiction.

Feeding the Brain What It Needs

- Whole and fresh foods (preferably organic) should constitute a healthy diet. Processed and sugary foods should be avoided.

- Three servings a day of good-quality protein (fish, poultry, lean free-range meat, eggs, soya or combinations of beans, lentils, and grains).

- Complex carbohydrates such as wholegrains, vegetables, and most fruits.

- Fish should be eaten at least three times a week, or fish oil supplements should be taken.

- Drink at least one or two litres of water per day, either pure or in diluted juices, herbal and fruit teas.

- Limit the intake of caffeinated tea, coffee, and soft drinks.

- At least five servings a day of antioxidant-rich fruit and vegetables (leeks, onions, garlic, eggplant, grapes, berries, pumpkin, mangoes, apricots, carrots, spinach, parsley).

Genetics

The genes which cause dementia and Alzheimer's disease have been identified as chromosomes #1, #12, #14, #19, #21, apolipoprotein C1 (and, more rarely, apolipoprotein E4 – a gene carried by only 30% of people, only 10% of whom develop Alzheimer's disease) and the HLA 2A gene. The younger a person is when they develop Alzheimer's disease, the more likely it is that it has been caused by genetic factors, particularly through the mother's linkage. Interestingly, the Cherokee native Americans appear to have natural resistance to the disease, while African Americans and Hispanics have a higher rate of it.

In order to understand how genetics works, we need to understand the basic structure of the human genome. In human beings, diploid sperm, and egg cells each have 23 chromosomes. One of these is a sex chromosome which determines the gender of the foetus (either X or Y). The genes are located in the chromosomes and are composed of highly ordered DNA. Capping the end of each chromosome is a telomere, a specialised structure made of DNA and protein, whose function is to prevent abnormality or loss of genetic information during cell division, which is the process of human growth. If the telomeres are shortened, they may no longer be able to support normal division of the chromosomes inside the cells. The result is abnormal chromosomal function, which can result in dysfunctional genes, a dysfunctional immune system, ageing of tissues and the development of cancer and chronic diseases.

Why would the telomeres become shortened? Because this happens with age. Also, some people start off with longer telomeres than others. In healthy cells, the gene that controls telomere "expression" (i.e., extension) is "silenced" – i.e., inactive.

TELOMERE

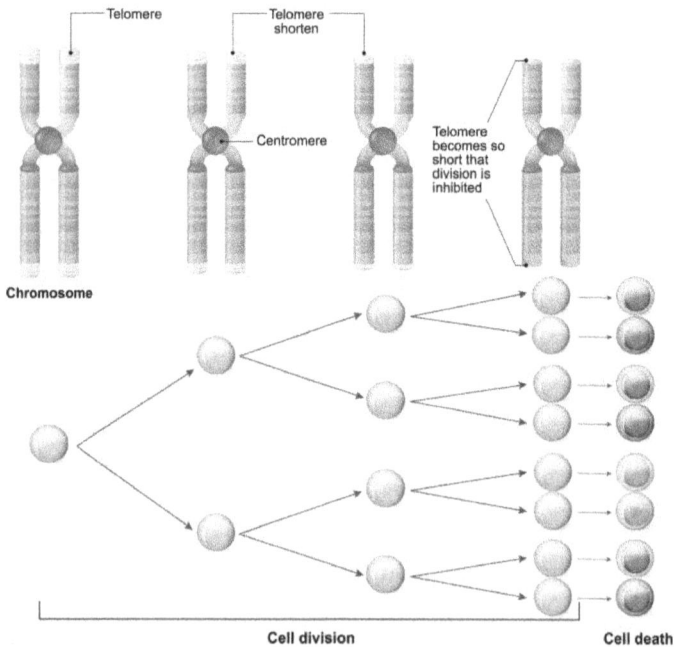

Thanks to genetic manipulation and the administration of certain compounds, it may be possible – to some extent – to "silence" this gene. What we know is that other factors, such as a sedentary lifestyle, oxidative stress, cancer, insulin-resistance (metabolic syndrome X and Type 2 diabetes) and chronic inflammatory disease, can all stunt telomere length. In addition, the length of telomeres is determined by gender (they are longer in women), age (they are longer in children), age of parents (older parents may deviate shorter telomeres to their offspring), menopause and andropause.

Of course, while leading a healthy lifestyle, becoming aware of our particular genetic profiles, and addressing the risks as far as possible are all important measures to take, the fact remains that genetic behaviour is largely beyond our control. A gene which develops a sequence variation (known as a polymorphism or mutation) can be inherited from a parent, or from an antecedent several generations before that, and unexpectedly begin to have an adverse effect on biological functioning, causing a "genetic disease". Likewise, a polymorphism may occur and have no effect at all on an individual. It is, in fact, very much like a lottery.

The most common polymorphisms are single nucleotide ones (SNPs, pronounced "snips"), which may have arisen many generations previously and been transmitted slowly among different populations (e.g., Tay-Sachs disease, thalassaemia, cystic fibrosis, Down's syndrome, haemophilia, and sickle cell anaemia). In some cases, the penetrance (likelihood) of a SNP occurring which causes illness in an individual is influenced by lifestyle factors such as the amount of phenylalanine in their diet, obesity, smoking, alcohol and drug misuse, exposure to toxins and – crucially – chronic inflammation. Healing from chronic inflammation is, in turn, influenced by age (the older the person, the slower the healing), deficiencies of nutrients such as vitamin C, protein, zinc and fatty acids, metabolic diseases, certain drugs and polymorphisms that result in higher basal levels of inflammatory agents.

Type 2 diabetes, hypertension, hypercholesterolaemia and heart disease all share a common genetic variation associated with the way the body uses insulin to metabolise sugars. This resistance to insulin means that the cells are less able to remove glucose from the bloodstream. *Tumour necrosis factor* (a pro-inflammatory cytokine (peptide)) is secreted by inflammatory cells and plays an important role in cell survival, proliferation, differentiation, and death – in other words, the development of cancer. The tumour necrosis factor gene may also be a marker for obesity and diabetes.

Similarly, the apolipoprotein carries lipoproteins, fat-soluble vitamins, and cholesterol into the lymph system. It also co-ordinates the transportation of lipids necessary for the formation of myelin, the protective nerve covering which is essential for brain plasticity and learning. However, the *Apo*

E4 genetic variation in that protein may make an individual 10% more likely to develop high cholesterol levels, 40% more likely to develop coronary heart disease and twice as likely to develop Alzheimer's disease. They are also likelier to take longer to recover from brain injuries or bleeds. Controlling the risks of Apo E4 is best done by dietary intervention, weight management, avoiding or limiting alcohol consumption and certain medications. Detoxification by administering phase II enzymes such as glutathione S-transferase (GST) is essential for strengthening cellular defence and reducing their susceptibility to carcinogens, especially in people who have the GSTM1 and GSTT1 null genetic polymorphism. The cells can be further protected by increasing the consumption (five to seven times a week) of cruciferous (crunchy) vegetables such as broccoli, cabbage, and cauliflower, as well as onions and garlic. Fried foods, grilled or roasted red meats, and smoked or cured meat, chicken or fish should be avoided.

Other genes, by contrast, are highly *beneficial*. The catechol O-methyltransferase (COMT) gene is responsible for the production of enzymes that counteract toxins associated with oxidative DNA damage. However, if the gene undergoes variation, prolonged exposure to the estrogen it produces may increase the risk of breast and prostate cancer. So, we see that some genes have both harmful and healing potential.

Diabetes is another disease in which genetics may play a role. While insufficient insulin is common to both Type 1 (an absolute deficiency of insulin) and Type 2 (a relative deficiency), 60-80% of Type 2 diabetics have the so-called "metabolic syndrome", meaning that there is a cluster of factors putting them at risk not just of diabetes, but also of cardiovascular disease due to hypertension, dyslipidemia (a lack of lipids in the blood, increasing the risk of clogged arteries, heart attack, stroke and other potentially fatal illnesses, especially in smokers, sedentary and obese people) and microalbuminuria (an increase of albumin in the urine, which could be a marker for kidney disease). Type 2 diabetes affects about 150 million people around the world and that number is predicted to double by the year 2036, with increasing numbers of younger people developing the disease. In the USA, Type 2 diabetes is now classified as an epidemic. Although lifestyle factors such as an unhealthy diet, lack of exercise, obesity and alcohol consumption have a lot to do with this, there is also evidence that the disease is highly prevalent among groups of people with a traditional lifestyle who emigrated to a more highly Westernised environment (e.g. Aboriginal Australians who have moved to the cities, Polynesian islanders who emigrated to New Zealand, Chinese who moved to Mauritius, Hong Kong, Singapore and Taiwan, Asian Indians who moved to Mauritius, Fiji, South Africa and the UK, as well as Yemenite

Jews who emigrated to Israel). It has been estimated that the diabetes risk in those with one diabetic parent is 40%, while a sibling of someone with Type 2 diabetes has a three times higher risk of developing the disease than others in the population.

The Calpain 10 and inwardly rectifying potassium channel Kir 6.2 (KCNJ11) genes increase susceptibility to Type 2 diabetes. Peroxisome proliferator-activated receptor-ɣ (PPARɣ) and a more common variant, Pro12AIa, are genes which mediate high-fat-induced obesity, lower the body mass index, increase insulin sensitivity, and lower the risk for diabetes. However, if PPARɣ undergoes a rare Pro115GIn mutation, it increases the cellular accumulation of triglycerides and the likelihood of morbid obesity. Similarly, the peroxisome proliferator-activated receptor-gamma coactivator-1 (PGC-1) is a key determinant for the development of slow-twitch muscle fibre, while the PGC-1α gene is reduced in the skeletal muscle, pancreas and possibly the liver of those with early Type 2 diabetes. These findings all suggest that inherited defects in mitochondrial genes could be significant contributors to the development of diabetes.

Adiponectin (APM1) – a protein hormone encoded in the ADIPOQ gene and produced mainly in adipose (fatty) tissue, as well as in muscle and the brain – helps to reduce glucose levels and heighten insulin sensitivity in the body. However, in individuals with obesity, Type 2 diabetes and cardiovascular disease, plasma levels of APM1 are reduced. Thus, we see the relationships between genes and lifestyle in determining whether diseases develop which, through a series of metabolic chain reactions in the body over time, could result in cognitive decline.

We are certain that this very intricate explanation has, once more, cowed our readers. However, take heart: the section is merely intended to explain (in admittedly arcane terms) the genetic influences which form part of the composite metabolic picture.

The most important learning of all this is that simply having the gene which predisposes one towards a particular disease does not necessarily mean one will develop it. Following a diet low in carbohydrates, cholesterol, saturated and trans fats and high in Omega-3 fatty acids, as well as getting at least 30-60 minutes of exercise three or four times a week, having regular blood pressure checks and managing stress levels can successfully prevent the onset of genetically favoured illnesses, most of which predispose a person to developing cognitive decline later in life. So, we are by no means at the mercy of destiny. There is much we can do to control our own health.

Head Trauma and Epilepsy

A traumatic head or brain injury, especially one involving a loss of consciousness, doubles the risk of Alzheimer's disease.

If the person suffering such an injury or loss of consciousness carries the apolipoprotein E4 gene *(see above)*, their risk of developing Alzheimer's increases tenfold. There is also increasing research linking seizure-like activities in the brain, as experienced by epileptics, with the kind of cognitive decline seen in Alzheimer's patients.

Diabetes and Hyperglycaemia

Increasing evidence is being found linking Type 2 diabetes to Alzheimer's disease. The diabetic brain is susceptible to neurodegenerative disease, as glucose (sugar) can cause changes in the body's proteins. Cyclo-oxygenase-2 (COX-2) – an enzyme that speeds up the production of certain chemical "messengers", called prostaglandins – can promote inflammation. In hyperglycaemia (as it is experienced in Type 2 diabetes), COX-2 and its inflammatory effects are increased. Diabetes can also lead to atrophy of the brain.

Gut Imbalance

An imbalance of the gut organisms (presenting as diarrhoea, cramps, flatulence, indigestion, constipation, bloating and irritability) can affect memory.

Anti-Diuretic Hormone (Hdh)

This is a condition in which a person is unable to retain water, leading to frequent urination. They may also have higher than normal salt levels on the skin, lower back pain, fungal overgrowth, depression, a tendency to allergies, obesity, frequent headaches, and other symptoms associated with chronic dehydration.

Iron

As a person ages, iron accumulates in their brain. According to recent research, this can contribute to memory decline and Alzheimer's disease, because when iron reacts with oxygen and water in our environment, it forms rust. Similarly, when iron levels in the body become too high, they trigger oxidation (the production of highly toxic free radicals, which damage and, ultimately, kill cells). Excess iron also contributes to the formation of brain plaques and tau protein tangles. High levels of iron in the brain have been found to impact the hippocampus, in particular – a key memory area.

Infections

Infections in any part of the body cause chronic inflammation, which plays an important part in the development of Alzheimer's disease. (In fact, Type 1 Alzheimer's is properly known as "inflammatory Alzheimer's disease"). The most common causes of infections are:

- the **herpes simplex virus type 1 (HSV1),** which is present in most of the population by the time they are 70. It travels to the brain in middle age, where it remains in a latent state until it is re-activated by events such as immunosuppression, peripheral infections, or inflammation. The consequent damage can eventually lead to Alzheimer's disease.

- **multiple antibiotic-resistant coagulase negative staphylococci (MARCoNS),** which reside deep in the nasal passage of 80% of people with low melanocyte-stimulating hormones (MSH), as well as in those who have been exposed to mould, had Lyme disease or biotoxin illnesses. These hormones are produced by the pituitary gland, hypothalamus and skin cells and are essential for protecting the skin from ultraviolet rays, the development of pigmentation and control of appetite. In individuals with low MSH levels, the body initially increases its levels of cortisol (a hormone produced by stress) to respond to the deficiency. However, if the body cannot sustain its cortisol production, adrenal fatigue sets in.

- MARCoNS is not actually an infection, but a colonisation of bacteria which can become one. The bacteria send chemicals into the blood which increase inflammation, causing a further drop in MSH levels. This, in turn, creates further inflammation.

- Lyme disease, which is caused by ticks (typically carried by dogs, cats, horses, and other animals) and manifests as a red rash about a week after one has been bitten. Left untreated, an infected bite eventually causes severe headaches, neck stiffness and red rashes on other parts of the body. There may be chronic fatigue, facial palsy, severe arthritic pain and swelling (especially in the knees and other large joints), pain in the tendons, muscles, joints and bones, heart palpitations, dizziness, shortness of breath, numbness and tingling in the hands and feet and, finally, inflammation of the spinal cord and brain.

- Intestinal dysbiosis, or microbial imbalance in the stomach, which can lead to "leaky gut" and may be linked to irritable bowel syndrome and Crohn's disease.

- biotoxin illness.

- chronic inflammatory response syndrome.

- chronic fatigue (symptoms typically include debilitating exhaustion and body aches) and immune dysfunction syndrome.

- Helicobacter pylori, bacteria which live in the gastric mucosa and the mouth (usually in dental plaque) and always cause inflammation. They are transmitted orally, through an infected person's saliva (e.g., through kissing). These are the most prevalent bacteria infecting humans in the world. The condition only has toxic effects in some people (about half of whom are aged over 50 and about 20% of whom are aged under 40), and is uncommon in young children. The infection is detected by means of a blood test, a breath test, a biopsy during an endoscopy, or a stool antigen test. Helicobacter pylori increase the risk of gingivitis and periodontal disease, atherosclerosis, abnormal blood clotting, ischaemic heart disease, stroke, gastritis, heartburn, migraine, rosacea (a red skin rash) and abdominal pain caused by indigestion. It may also increase the risk of Alzheimer's disease and Guillain-Barré syndrome. The bacteria can interfere with the body's amino acids, digestive system chemicals, peptides, and levels of vitamin B12.

- periodontal disease, which occurs when bacteria infect the gum tissue surrounding teeth. The infection slowly erodes the surrounding structure, causing teeth to lose bone and ligament support. Abscesses may form and the area becomes swollen and extremely painful. In most cases, extraction of the tooth is required and/ or an apisectomy (a surgical procedure in which a filling is inserted at the tip of the tooth root and the surrounding infected tissue removed). Periodontal disease is caused by poor dental hygiene (not brushing or flossing teeth regularly), smoking, lack of regular dental cleaning and genetic predisposition. It is associated with Alzheimer's disease and can also exacerbate heart conditions, as the swelling of tissue increases plaque build-up, which may inflame the arteries.

- cytomegalovirus, a member of the herpes virus family which affects 60-99% of adults worldwide.

- heat shock proteins (formed when cells are briefly exposed to temperatures above their normal growth temperature). Despite their name, they can also be formed during exposure to cold, ultraviolet light and during wound-healing or tissue-remodelling. In genetically predisposed people, the antibodies to these proteins may also accelerate atherosclerosis.

- yeast infections or Candida albicans, which is one of 70 different species of candida yeast that develops in the mouth, oesophagus, intestines, or vagina. It is caused by the consumption and fermentation of sucrose and other simple sugars and, left untreated, can proliferate to the entire system (particularly in immunosuppressed individuals such as HIV/Aids patients or those undergoing chemotherapy). When this occurs, it changes from a yeast-fungal form to a mycelial-fungal form that produces rhizoids (long, root-like components that can pierce the walls of the intestinal tract that protect the intestines from blood). This may cause allergic reactions which, in turn, can break the blood-brain barrier. Systemic candidiasis can also affect the liver, kidney and brain and usually involves bloating, itching and rashes. The factors causing candida to become systemic include a high intake of milk or lactose, alcohol, cheese, peanuts, dried fruit, mushrooms, potatoes and sweet potatoes, melons, figs, apricots, milk or lactose intake, certain drugs (e.g., steroids, birth control pills, synthetic estrogen and antibiotics), liver function impairment, nutrient deficiencies, and menstrual cycle hormone changes (e.g., during menopause).

- Other forms of candidiasis include *superficial candidiasis* (affecting areas of the skin and mucous membranes, including the toes and fingers, nailbeds, groin, mouth, and vagina). Clinical testing is needed for diagnosis. *Mucocutaneous candidiasis* is a serious infection which is associated with genetic malfunction of the white blood cells.

Chronic or Systemic Illnesses

- **Multiple sclerosis** is a condition in which the body's auto-immune system attacks the myelin sheaths on the nerves, causing progressive loss of communication between the brain and the rest of the body. It most often affects young adults and is a severe inflammatory disease.

- **Epstein-Barr virus** is an extremely common disease, affecting up to 95% of the human population worldwide. It hides inside the white blood cells and remains relatively dormant for the host's entire lifetime. However, if the immune system is unable to control it, it can be re-activated, causing tumours. It has been repeatedly associated with multiple sclerosis and other auto-immune diseases.

- **Atherosclerotic disease** (hardening and/or narrowing of the arteries), caused by a build-up of fats, cholesterol, and other substances in and on the artery walls (plaque), thus restricting blood flow. If the plaque bursts, it causes a blood clot to form, which can lead to a stroke. While atherosclerosis is most often associated with the heart, it can affect arteries anywhere in the body. Research has shown that Helicobacter pylori, the herpes simplex virus and the cytomegalovirus are all involved in triggering atherosclerotic disease.

- **Attention deficit disorder (ADD).** While this is a condition distinct from Alzheimer's disease, they have many similarities and can both lead to dementia. ADD, like Alzheimer's, is a multi-factorial condition, caused by genetic factors, exposure to environmental toxins (air pollution, fertilisers, pesticides), toxins such as mercury, nutrient insufficiency, traumatic head injury, stress, food allergies, intestinal parasites, chronic infections, and an imbalance in the biochemical mediators dopamine (which regulates movement and mood), serotonin and norepinephrine.

- **Pyroluria (pyrrole disorder)** is a stress-related condition which depletes the body of certain vitamins and minerals before they can be absorbed, primarily vitamin B6, magnesium and zinc. The symptoms of the condition include sensitivity to sunlight and cold weather, tremors or spasms, inability to eat in the early morning, nausea, abdominal pain, severe headaches, rapid pulse, nervous exhaustion, extreme emotions (excitability, depression), fear of mingling with others or becoming dependent on family and insomnia.

- **Vitamin B6 deficiency** can be diagnosed by a patient's inability to recall dreams.

STAGES OF COGNITIVE DECLINE

There are seven identified stages of cognitive decline in Alzheimer's disease, ranging in severity. Stages 1-6 are reversible with the correct treatment, based on the patient's particular medical history, lifestyle, age, and circumstances. Stage 7 is too advanced to be reversed, but is still manageable, depending on the doctor's level of monitoring and the patient's level of compliance.

Stage 1

This is the mildest form of Alzheimer's at its onset, when its effects are still barely perceptible. There is no significant memory loss, and no signs of dementia are evident.

Stage 2

Very mild decline, when the patient may experience minor lapses of memory (e.g., forgetting where they left things), but no more than normal age-related memory loss. The patient can still function well and neither their family nor doctor is likely to detect the condition. Short-term memory loss is likely to improve with mind exercises. However, the memory retrieval mechanism naturally slows down with age.

Stage 3

Mild decline. The family members and doctor become aware of significant cognitive problems, including aphasia (forgetting words and names, or forgetting something they have just read), inability to arrange or organise, as well as a tendency to lose personal items, including valuables. This stage of the disease generally lasts about seven years prior to the onset of dementia and it is the ideal time for the person to attend to legal, financial, and other important matters, while they are still able to participate meaningfully in decision-making.

Stage 4

Moderate decline, where the disease becomes clearly evident. The person can no longer do simple calculations (e.g., budget or manage money correctly), forgets what they did or said that morning and cannot recall certain details in their histories (e.g., where they once lived or friends they once had). This stage usually lasts about two years.

Stage 5

Moderately severe decline. At this stage of the disease, patients can no longer perform certain day-to-day activities, such as dressing appropriately, remembering their phone number, or distinguishing between days. They may still be able to bath and use the toilet unaided, recognise family members and may recall surprisingly detailed – and obscure - events from their early childhood or youth, but not more recent ones. On average, this stage lasts about 18 months.

Stage 6

Severe decline. The patient's condition now poses the risk of injury, since they are unaware of their surroundings, become prone to wandering off and forgetting where they live, can no longer use the toilet or bath without assistance, lose control of their bladder and bowel, and recognise only their closest friends and relatives. This is also the stage where they may undergo a significant personality change, becoming aggressive, paranoid, argumentative or very withdrawn. They may also exhibit compulsive, repetitive behaviour, such as handwringing or tissue-shredding. They have no insight into their own condition, apart from occasional, brief flashes of lucidity. This stage usually lasts for about two-and-a-half years and is typically the point at which families seek institutionalised geriatric care for the patient.

Stage 7

Very severe decline. This is the final stage of Alzheimer's disease, where patients who are left untreated are approaching death. They can no longer communicate or respond to their environment. They may retain the ability to utter certain words or phrases, but these are often inappropriate to where they are. Nevertheless, they may still respond to gentle touching or relaxing music. They must be helped with all essential activities, including eating, and may lose the ability to walk, sit unaided or swallow, requiring them to be fed intravenously and possibly catheterised. They also become vulnerable to infections, especially pneumonia. This stage of the illness can no longer be reversed. However, with the correct treatment, it may be arrested and managed. The patient is completely unaware of their own condition. This stage lasts about two-and-a-half years.

Given this trajectory, then, we see that Alzheimer's disease is a progressive illness which gradually deteriorates over a period lasting four to 20 years. In most cases, patients live four to eight years after diagnosis, depending on their genetic profile, medical history, lifestyle, and circumstances.

Treatment Of
Cognitive Decline

A S WITH OTHER CONDITIONS considered to be "dread diseases" and stigmatised for that reason, a tragically high number of Alzheimer's disease (cognitive decline) patients do not seek medical care until extremely late in the development of the illness. Most of them are misinformed and believe nothing can be done to help them – that it is simply a matter of "waiting for the inevitable end". They fear that in the immediate term, their lifestyles will be severely impacted by having their driver's licences revoked and that in the longer term, they will be unable to afford private care or nursing home placement. Families, for their part, are equally afraid of such a diagnosis, preferring to live in denial as long as possible. Both these perceptions are largely the result of the stigmatisation of Alzheimer's disease as an incurable and intensely traumatic condition for which there is neither relief nor remedy.

Similarly, primary care providers (doctors) often fail to refer Alzheimer's patients for specialised treatment because they, too, believe that it is an essentially irremediable condition. In many cases, they simply start patients presenting with cognitive decline on donepezil (Aricept) without even doing a firm diagnosis.

And specialists (neurologists, etc), for their part, frequently put patients through hours of neuropsychological testing, expensive imaging, lumbar punctures, and other procedures, but still have little or nothing to offer therapeutically.

However, the primary reason conventional medicine has failed so badly at curing Alzheimer's disease is that specialists expect to find a single, enormous, pharmaceutical monotherapy which can address *all* facets of the disease in *all* patients, at *all* stages of the spectrum. This does not – and will never – exist, since it is a multi-faceted condition requiring a multi-faceted therapeutic approach.

DIAGNOSIS

Ideally, the approach of the doctor should be a **functional integrative** one. The doctor needs to understand the biochemical, mental, emotional, spiritual, and athletic/recreational individuality of that particular patient, and the elements which created or impacted that composite profile. The functionality of the patient's eliminatory system (i.e., the body's ability to detoxify itself) and their defence and repair systems (i.e., preventing and restoring damage) must also be understood. A person in their 60s or 70s who leads a sedentary lifestyle, eats a diet high in cholesterol and low in protein, is largely reclusive and gets no more than four or five hours' sleep a night because of depression is likely to have a vastly different profile from someone the same age who takes daily exercise, has an active social life, eats wholesome foods and is an avid reader, thus receiving regular mental stimulation.

When diagnosing Alzheimer's disease, the doctor needs to ask: **"From what is the patient's brain protecting itself?"** Inflammation? Infection? Oral bacteria? Fungi or moulds? A leaky gut or blood-brain barrier? Toxins such as metals? He or she should obtain a clear picture of the patient's whole medical history, particularly triggering factors that may have precipitated the condition (such as head trauma, significant exposure to toxins, drug, or alcohol abuse, etc) and the mediators (factors that perpetuated the disease), from childhood to their current state. The patient's medical state must be carefully assessed and an understanding of their genetic profile, lifestyle and dietary habits obtained. Since all chronic illnesses have pathway imbalances which were signalled in the progression of the condition, these must be noted and balanced. The better the balance, the more positive the outcome of the Alzheimer's patient's treatment. It is essential that this is done **before** the doctor begins reducing the amyloids (plaque) in the brain, since the cause of the plaque building up must be addressed first.

HLA Typing

HLA typing is a genetic test use to identify certain individual variations in person's immune system. This is often the first step in assessing a person's susceptibility to Alzheimer's disease. Those who possess one or more of the 10 identified genotypes (the genetic factors associated with the condition) are less likely to be able to clear tiny toxins and inflammagens inhaled from mould and bacteria in damp environments, and may be unable to produce sufficient antigens (the substances which cause the immune system to recognise and fight off attacks from toxins and infections by producing antibodies).

Diagnosing Mould Infections

The doctor needs to ask the patient whether they live or work in a building with leaks, a damp basement, humidity problems, condensation on the windows, musty odours, discoloured wall and ceiling tiles or plaster. The patient should also be asked whether they developed their condition after moving to a new home, got a new job in a different location or began spending time in a new environment (church, gym, etc).

The diagnosis of Lyme disease is most often done with the Western blot (molecular analysis to detect specific proteins) or polymerase chain reaction (PCR) antigen tests. Babesiosis (a rare and life-threatening infection of the red blood cells, spread by ticks) is diagnosed with blood smears in the early stages. In later stages, PCR tests and mapping of the genetic material in the cells may be done. Testing of vitamin B12 and magnesium levels should be done (clues to deficiencies include twitching, poor stamina, and muscle spasms), as should pituitary and adrenal hormone assessment, thyroid testing and scanning of the brain.

The physical examination of the patient should include vital signs to detect tachycardia (irregular heartbeat), the body mass index, the presence of low-grade fever, a pallid or grey appearance, the ability to maintain pupillary response for longer than 10 seconds, inflammation of the mouth or gums, furriness or discolouration of the tongue, an enlarged thyroid, wheezing, bowel sounds, bladder tenderness, skeletal or postural weakness, open lesions on the skin (especially the scalp), rashes on the chest or upper back, bruising, cold or blue fingers and toes and tremors with outstretched hands.

Visual contrast testing should be done – a procedure which measures the patient's ability to distinguish between finer and finer increases of light versus darkness.

The doctor should also note the emotional state of the patient – i.e., whether they are tearful or anxious.

The doctor needs to note which of the patient's **lifestyle factors** are modifiable, such as their diet, exercise routine, exposure to toxins, usage of narcotics and alcohol, and whether they are getting sufficient sleep. Immunorestoration and detoxification of the lymphatic system both take place during sleep. Exercise is essential for both physical and brain health, and keeping the body moving and doing brain exercises are important in treating cognitive degeneration.

The patient's stress levels are another important consideration. Cortisol (the "stress hormone") can cause shrinkage of the brain, loss of memory, hormonal imbalances, and immunosuppression. Relationships, emotional and spiritual well-being are vital in controlling stress.

The patient's age and genetic profile also need to be considered, as the genes which cause Alzheimer's have been found to be chromosomes #1, #12, #14, #19, #21, apoliprotein C1 (and, more rarely, apolipoprotein E4) and the HLA 2A gene. The younger a patient is when the disease is diagnosed, the likelier it is that it was caused by hereditary factors, particularly through the mother's linkage.

The patient's gut health (the digestion and absorption of nutrients), energy production, biotransformation, detoxification, cardiovascular functioning, cellular communication and membrane health, endocrine levels, transmitters, structural integrity, assimilation, and mitochondrial membrane health are all metabolically active parts of the body, so a functional medicine matrix means that all these systems work together – none of them work alone. They form a web-like, overall system which must be balanced in order for the brain to receive the trophic support it requires. The patient's lifestyle, in turn, largely impacts this system and how balanced it is. A holistic approach – i.e., a **functional integrative medicine model** – is therefore needed in reaching a diagnosis of Alzheimer's, based on the overall metabolic health of the patient (and what he or she may have done, or be doing, to undermine it), and in treating it.

Laboratory Testing

There are numerous laboratory tests used to detect the reasons for cognitive decline, especially when other tests have failed in patients who are continually fatigued and not responding to supplements. An **Oligo-Lab** test – which is done using a hand-held device called a spectrophotometer, positioned briefly over points of the patient's palm – records the wavelengths of minerals and metals in the cells of tissues. This information is then transmitted to a web application in a cloud, where it is processed and analysed. Seconds later, the results appear on the doctor's computer screen, where it can then be used to draw up a treatment plan including the patient's nutrition, lifestyle, and supplements.

The intracellular information provided by Oligo-Lab tests is far more difficult to obtain through conventional blood and urine tests, though these are still important for obtaining measures for other things. By analysing the content of cellular tissue, an Oligo-Lab test shows a patient's metabolism and homeostasis (the state of their internal physical and chemical condition), as well as the concentration of toxic metals present which are undermining their health.

Common laboratory tests may also be conducted to measure blood count and chemistry, lipid, and hormone levels, as well as detect the presence of infectious diseases which cause inflammation. Stool analysis and tests to determine the patient's energy production and detoxification markers are important to give the doctor a composite picture of the patient's entire metabolic functioning.

A test for **histamine,** a major brain transmitter, is essential. Histamine stimulates the release of serotonin and norepinephrine, and also releases and balances dopamine. A *low* level of it in the blood (histapenia) means the patient is likely to have a depressed metabolism and is over-methylating (i.e., adding methyl groups onto other chemical compounds so that the body's processes can function properly. Methylation is a biochemical process similar to flicking on a switch to activate the repair of damaged DNA, produce energy, regulate hormones, detoxify the body, synthesise neurotransmitters, etc. Both over- and under-methylating cause this "switch" to be faulty.) Histapenic people are typically pear-shaped, with an accumulation of fat around the lower abdomen and thighs. Over-methylated people may also be prone to anxiety and manic or delusional psychological conditions and may suffer from canker sores (small, shallow sores in the mouth), inability to experience orgasm, hirsutism, and food sensitivities. They have high levels of copper, which is linked to psychotic behaviour, and may experience tinnitus (ringing in the ears), stuttering, weight increase and a tendence to abuse alcohol or recreational drugs.

Conversely, *high* levels of histamine in the blood (histadelia) mean the patient is under-methylating, has a fast metabolism and is using up nutrients too quickly. This is caused by a lack of B6, as well as stomach bugs, ingested histamine and high estrogen levels, all of which elevate histamine. The excess histamine is stored in the brain, which then disrupts the release of serotonin, dopamine, and norepinephrine, and becomes inflamed. As we know, serotonin and dopamine are the "feel-good" chemicals that promote a sense of well-being, while norepinephrine is responsible for memory, attention, and alertness. Low levels of any of these neurotransmitters can cause a person to exhibit aggression, hyperactivity, obsessive-compulsive behaviour, and exaggerated competitiveness. They may also become lachrymose and entertain suicidal thoughts. The physical symptoms include allergies, headaches, and increased sensitivity to pain. Histadelic people are typically of lean, slender build.

The causes of histadelia are thought to be genetic mutation, but it is likely that exposure to toxins and mould, high stress levels and nutrient deficiencies are also markers.

Saliva Testing for Adrenal Burnout

Saliva testing for adrenal burnout is usually done by taking three samples in the course of a day and evening. However, cortisone levels can falsely elevate the results.

24-Hour Urine Testing

24-hour urine testing for total hormonal output can provide a wealth of information regarding intracellular, hormonal and enzyme activity, while the cortisol levels in the urine indicate whether there is adrenal fatigue. The patient must be careful not to miss a void.

Pupil Test

A **"pupil"** test for adrenal fatigue is not necessarily done in a laboratory: it can be done at home. It is performed in a darkened room by shining a bright light from a steep angle into the patient's pupil. The normal pupillary reaction is to constrict and remain constricted. However, if the pupil dilates again (opens back up) after one to two minutes and takes another 30-45 seconds before constricting again, then the patient probably has a degree of adrenal fatigue.

Recent studies at the Mayo Clinic's Alzheimer's Disease Research Centre and the Mayo Clinic Study of Ageing in the USA have found that changes to the retina could fore-shadow Alzheimer's and Parkinson's diseases, as well as other neurodegenerative conditions. Pinched off from the brain during development in the uterus, the retina contains layers of neurons which researchers believe experience neurode-generation in tandem with their "cousins" inside the skull. The key difference is that these retinal neurons – which are located directly against the jelly-like, vitreous gel of the eyeball – are visible.

Researchers have found that by the time a patient first presents with memory problems or tremors, the neurode-generative process has probably been taking place for years – or even decades. Blood vessels have atrophied, neurons have died prematurely, and clumps of misfolded proteins have disrupted communication between them. Obviously, detecting these diseases early by retinal screening means being able to intervene early and prevent cognitive impair-ment. Moreover, retinal screening is non-invasive, less expensive than blood tests (and considerably less expensive than PET scans). Research indicates that it is also remark-ably sensitive, meaning it is also accurate.

Maya Koronyo-Hamaoui, a neuroscientist and professor of neurology at Cedars-Sinai in Los Angeles, California, USA, and her team have pioneered a technique to visualise the plaques associated with Alzheimer's disease in the retinal neurons of patients with mild (or early-stage) cognitive impairment. The patients are prepared for the procedure by loading up on protein shakes spiked heavily with curcumin, which has an extreme affinity for amyloid beta – the protein which makes up Alzheimer's plaques.

Another American biomedical pioneer – Dr Ruogu Fang, at the University of Florida – uses a fundus camera, a specialised iPhone attachment, to take high-resolution images of the microscopic blood vessels in the back of the eye. Changes to the blood vessels in the brain are characteristic of both Alzheimer's and Parkinson's diseases, due to premature neuron death, and researchers have compelling evidence that the blood vessels in the retina mirror those changes. Although the research is still new, initial results of computer algorithms using the fundus images suggest that they can distinguish Parkinson's patients from healthy control subjects with an accuracy of more than 70%. Although none of these biomarkers are perfect – since many people with elevated amyloid beta remain cognitively normal and vascular changes are also present in a myriad of other conditions, including diabetic retinopathy and traumatic brain injury – the research is highly encouraging for the early detection of neurodegenerative disease.

Sergent's White Line

The Sergent's White Line test (devised by Dr Emile Sergent in 1917) is done by lightly scraping the skin of the abdomen for a length of about 15cm. In a normal person, a red line should appear within seconds. The longer this red line takes to appear, the more severe the adrenal fatigue of the patient.

Hair Trace Mineral Analysis

Hair trace mineral analysis is a way of assessing the mineral balance in the body, which is crucial for maintaining health. A **mineral ratio** is basically assessed using the formula of one mineral level divided by a second one – a more accurate way of exposing nutritional deficiencies than analysing mineral levels alone. Mineral ratios show disease trends, which are predictive of future or hidden metabolic dysfunctions in the patient. The basic mineral ratios are **calcium/magnesium (blood-sugar),** for which the normal rate is 6,67:1. Calcium is needed for the pancreas to release insulin, while magnesium inhibits that secretion, so a balance is crucial. A very high or low imbalance is associated with mental and emotional disturbances.

Equally crucial is the **sodium/potassium** ratio, which can be life-threatening if it is out of kilter. Both sodium and potassium regulate the electric potential of cells (sodium extracellularly, potassium intracellularly). Their ratio is intricately linked to kidney, liver, and adrenal gland function, as well as immune system functioning. A high ratio can trigger asthma, allergies, renal and hepatic disorders. However, a low ratio is more dangerous, since it can result in cardiac failure, cancer, arthritis, kidney, and liver disorders. In assessing the sodium/potassium ratio, the doctor needs to bear in mind that the presence of mercury (cadmium toxicity) can influence the reading.

The **calcium/potassium ratio** is also called the **thyroid ratio,** as both calcium and potassium play a vital role in regulating thyroid activity. The ideal ratio is 4:1. A ratio less than this indicates increased thyroid activity (i.e., fast metabolism, marked by hyperactivity, irritability, excessive sweating, nervousness, oily hair, and skin, as well as diarrhoea (especially during times of stress)). A high ratio is exhibited by a tendency to gain weight, cold extremities, lack of sweating, fatigue, dry skin and hair, and constipation.

The **sodium/magnesium ratio** is obtained from a tissue reading, rather than a hair trace analysis. This is also called the adrenal ratio, since it is directly associated with the adrenal gland, which is a major regulator of the rate of metabolism. Aldosterone (a mineral corticoid adrenal hormone) regulates the retention of sodium in the system. The higher the sodium level, the higher the aldosterone level. The symptoms of under-active adrenal gland include exhaustion, depression, low blood sugar, weight fluctuations, poor digestion of fats and meat protein and allergies. An over-active adrenal gland is marked by a tendency to inflammation, high energy and drive, aggressiveness, impulsiveness, high blood pressure, diabetes, and a Type A personality (competitive, highly organised, impatient, focused, intolerant of mistakes, obsessive).

The **calcium/phosphorus ratio** should ideally be 1-2:1. In addition to magnesium and vitamin D, they are vital to bone health.

The **iron/copper ratio** is important in cellular respiration and electron transport.

The **zinc/copper ratio** is important for brain health. Both minerals are influenced by several physiological and hormonal factors, including estrogen, progesterone and testosterone.

Individuals who embark on nutritional balancing programmes based on hair mineral analysis frequently begin to eliminate excess copper. The reason is that deficiencies of zinc, manganese, and other minerals in the body result in an accumulation of copper in the tissues. However, free, or unbound copper can be toxic, since it is a powerful oxidant which can cause inflammation. To avoid toxicity, copper should be bound or wrapped in protein molecules. Sulphur amino acids (found in eggs and meat) can achieve this, while sufficient adrenal glandular activity is also necessary for the liver to produce copper-binding proteins.

When the body gets rid of excess copper, it is moved from tissue storage sites to the blood, which transports it to the liver and kidneys, through which it is eliminated. However, if this does not happen rapidly enough (i.e., if uncleared copper remains in the blood), the individual can experience headaches, anxiety, fatigue, skin rashes, testicular pain in men, changes in the menstrual cycle in women, irritability, and tearfulness – all symptoms which are unpleasant, but temporary.

One way of preventing this is by stopping the nutritional balancing programme for about three days, thus giving the body a break from the supplements. During this break, it is advisable to eat eggs or other animal protein regularly, while also drinking plenty of water. It is also helpful to take molybdenum, which binds with copper to reduce its toxic effects, Russian black radish (a herb high in sulphur, which helps with liver detoxification), N-acetyl cysteine, a compound equally rich in sulphur) and L-taurine (an essential amino acid which also helps bind and eliminate copper).

Other ways of relieving the symptoms of copper elimination are slow walking and deep breathing, which help calm the nerves and encourage the liver, kidneys, and intestines to remove copper, as well as taking one or two coffee enemas daily, which stimulate bile flow and enhance liver detoxification. The enema comprises 30mg of regular ground coffee dissolved in 500ml boiling water, which is then left to simmer for five minutes. Once the mixture cools to body temperature, it can be decanted into an enema bag. The enema should be retained for 15 minutes for maximum effectiveness.

Sauna baths and massages are also useful for decongesting the liver and kidneys, as are acupressure or acupuncture.

As with all other disorders, however, prevention is better than cure. Ideally, one should avoid copper build-up by limiting one's intake of seafood (oysters, crabs, bluefish, perch, and lobster), meats (veal, lamb, pork, beef liver and beef kidneys), duck, nuts (almonds, pecans, walnuts, Brazil nuts and pistachios), sesame and sunflower seeds, soybeans, wheatgerm and bran. One should also avoid prolonged exposure to copper water pipes, copper compounds used in swimming pools, copper cookware and kettles, copper jewellery and copper intra-uterine devices.

The **alpha-melanocyte-stimulating hormone (alpha-MSH)** is a crucial neuropeptide which is produced in the hypothalamus, the area of the brain that exercises hormonal control of the body and where the nervous system meets the endocrine system. Small amounts of alpha-MSH may also be produced in the brainstem. It regulates other hormones in the body, stimulates the release of endorphins, regulates inflammatory responses and is part of the innate immune system, e.g., by regulating the body's basic defences against microbes. It also regulates weight by reducing food intake and enables melanocytes to cause tanning of the skin.

Low levels of alpha-MSH cause chronic fatigue due to low cortisol and poor control of the thyroid hormones. Increased inflammation and reduced endorphin production result in pain, while the patient may experience severe sleep disorders, appetite swings, night sweats, poor regulation of body temperature, leaky gut, and susceptibility to microbial attack and biotoxin-related illness.

Telomere Testing

Initial telomere testing is offered by SpectraCell laboratories in Houston, Texas, USA, which provides a "telomere score" by measuring telomere length on T lymphocytes. This is calculated by comparing the measurements with results from the American population of the same age. However, this is an expensive and protracted procedure. There are other, far simpler (and more affordable) ways to prevent telomere shortening:

- Weight control.

- Stress reduction.

- Avoiding the abuse of substances such as simple sugar, tobacco, alcohol and illicit/recreational and unnecessary over the counter or prescription drugs.

- Optimum nutrition. *Dietary supplements* can support telomere structure and function, particularly ginkgo biloba, astragalus, Chinese ginger root, vitamins D3 and B12, folic acid, nicotinamide, Omega-3 fatty acids and multivitamins and/or antioxidants. In addition, a telomere-supporting diet should be low in carbohydrates, saturated fats and trans fatty acids, but high in dietary fibre (to counter insulin-resistance), comprising low-calorie, nutrient-dense foods, plenty of fruit and vegetables, and a balanced intake (no more than 1g per kilogram of body weight per day) of rotated protein from lean meat, cold-water fish, and dairy products. In addition, there should be intermittent short periods of fasting and detoxification.

- Management of diseases such as cardiovascular disease (atherosclerosis), hypertension, diabetes, and metabolic syndrome X, which are classic disorders causing premature ageing. This is done by ensuring that blood sugar levels and blood pressure are maintained at the correct levels, reducing chronic inflammation, controlling weight, and embarking on an exercise programme as part of one's permanent lifestyle.

Treating
Alzheimer's Disease

ALZHEIMER'S IS NOT INCURABLE. Such a notion is old-school. Nowadays there are tools at our disposal to diagnose the different causes of the condition and how to treat it.

The correct approach is one which is patient-centred, holistic and strives to achieve a dynamic balance of internal (metabolic) and external (lifestyle) factors. It is important to remember that health is not defined as merely the absence of disease, but as quality of life and joy – a positive vitality. The treatment of Alzheimer's should aim to restore to the patient confidence, cognitive functioning, and the ability to participate in their surroundings and engage with others meaningfully.

As we have explained, the approach of the treating doctor should be one of **integrative medicine,** focusing not on the endpoint of a treatment or a pathological state, but on the dynamic processes which came before it and resulted in the condition. In other words, it should seek a path of therapy which includes all those preceding elements and addresses the underlying **causes,** both metabolic and external, rather than just the symptoms of the disease (forgetfulness, confusion, disorientation, etc).

Ideally, a full battery of laboratory blood tests (both conventional and functional), as well as testing of chronic inflammatory response syndrome, immune function, hormone levels, gut function, a Dutch test analysis, GI map testing, testing for AoeE4 (the gene most associated with the eventual development of Alzheimer's disease), methylation testing, neurotransmitter testing, microbiome and Viome testing (of the gut microbiome) should be done. This gives the doctor a comprehensive profile of the patient's physiological history and predispositions.

The doctor should then do a full enquiry of the patient's environment, lifestyle, level of education (i.e., their awareness and/or understanding of maintaining wellness), psychological and emotional state. An assessment of the patient's skills and abilities linked to brain function (i.e., attention span, problem-solving, memory, language, IQ, visual-spatial and academic skills) is also necessary, as this will help determine the patient's level of cognitive functioning. The results of these assessments can be compared with the outcomes of later tests (which should be done periodically), in order to indicate the rate of decline.

Once the doctor has a clear understanding of which contributors have caused amyloid plaque to build up in the brain, and has prioritised a personalised treatment regimen addressing all those factors, treatment should continue until improvement begins. This can take several months, and regular monitoring is crucial.

What is required in treating Alzheimer's disease is a multi-modality approach of combined interventions. No single agent is likely to be effective. Drugs are the "dessert" of the treatment, not the entrée.

Hormone replacement can produce remarkable results in Type 2 dementia.

Colystyrene (a bowel acid) is used to manage cholesterol levels, while binders such as cholestyramine, clay, charcoal, chlorella, etc can help to bind mould.

Saunas can help to release dirt, while Bactroban (mupirocin) – a topical antibiotic – and colloidal silver (a natural antimicrobial agent) can be used to strengthen the immune system. These treatments are generally prescribed for about four weeks.

NUTRITIONAL AND LIFESTYLE CHANGES
The Ketogenic Diet

Medical research indicates that one of the most effective lifestyle changes to make in preventing and treating cognitive decline is the adoption of a ketogenic diet. This is a diet which is low in carbohydrates (10%), moderate in protein (20%) and high in fat (70%). This causes the body to burn fat for energy, rather than glucose, resulting in the production of ketone bodies (molecules that can be used as a source of fat).

Ketones are by-products of the breakdown of fat for fuel in the body. In a healthy (non-diabetic) person, insulin, glucagon, and other hormones prevent ketone levels from becoming too high (1,6-3,0 mmol/L). The desirable level is 0,6-1,6 mmol/L. These levels can be measured in the urine, blood, and breath. The brain and other organs and tissues rely on ketones as a source of energy.

The most effective way of keeping ketone levels at a moderate level is by lowering one's intake of carbohydrates (ideally, to no more than 50g per day) and increasing one's intake of fats. Fewer carbohydrates help promote the breakdown of fats and shift the body into ketosis. Certain patients – e.g., those with inborn metabolic disorders, Type 1 diabetes, kidney or liver disease – may be advised to increase their intake of ketones through nutritional supplements ("exogenous" ketones), rather than through a modification of their daily eating habits ("endogenous" ketones).

Other patients may be advised by their doctors to follow a ketogenic diet only for a specific period of weeks or months, or to follow it cyclically (i.e., for shorter periods a few times a year).

For those able to undertake long-term eating modification, a ketogenic diet – like all sustainable food regimens – should be one which becomes part of their permanent lifestyle, not a temporary "break" before returning to unhealthy eating. After embarking on a ketogenic diet, it typically takes a few days for the body to adjust to using fat as an energy source, rather than glucose. During this period, many people experience a feeling similar to withdrawal from toxins, called "keto flu", with dizziness, drowsiness, mild body aches, nausea, or irritability. There may also be cramping, stomach pains and muscle tenderness. Drinking more water, eating quality fat (e.g., fatty salmon), taking a ketonic supplement, getting more exercise and plenty of sleep help to mitigates these symptoms. Within seven to 14 days, they subside, and a significant improvement is usually noticeable.

The reason ketogenic diets are important is that as we age, our brains – which rely solely on glucose for energy when we are young and healthy – are less able to do so. A reduction of 10-16% of glucose uptake is typical in healthy, older individuals, while a reduction of as much as 35% can be experienced in those with neurological diseases such as Alzheimer's disease or other conditions causing cognitive decline. It is therefore crucial to provide the brain with an alternative source of energy, since it cannot use free fatty acids, which come from saturated, mono-unsaturated, polyunsaturated and trans fats.

These unhealthy, free fatty acids are typically found in butter, ghee, suet, lard, coconut and palm oil, cakes, biscuits and other confections, fatty meat (lamb, mutton, boerewors), cured or smoked meats such as bacon, ham, sausages, salami, chorizo and pancetta, cheese, pastries, cream (including sour cream and crème fraîche, ice cream, coconut milk and coconut cream), milkshakes, chocolate, and chocolate spreads.

There are also other significant benefits to a ketogenic diet. Weight loss is one, since a diet which is rich in fat and low in carbohydrates eliminates the need for the body to break down muscle protein into glucose. And that, in turn, decreases the blood sugar and insulin levels. The result is an increase in the metabolism of fatty acids.

In patients with cognitive decline, allowing the brain to stop using glucose for energy encourages greater nerve growth and synaptic connections between brain cells. The patient is therefore more alert, with improved focus and cognitive capabilities. And in patients with diabetes, a low-carbohydrate diet helps support insulin metabolism in the body, so that more insulin is circulating and contributing to glucose control.

Some have expressed concerns about the advisability of following a diet high in fat because of rising cholesterol levels. However, a ketogenic diet is designed to increase primarily high-density lipoprotein (HDL, or "good") cholesterols and reduce "bad" low-density lipoprotein (LDL) or very-low-density lipoprotein (VLDL) cholesterol. With regular monitoring of the patient's blood lipid profile, waist circumference, inflammation, insulin signalling, blood sugar levels and lean body mass, there should be no significant cholesterol risk.

It is not only the medical fraternity who are aware of the benefits of a ketogenic diet. Athletes and professional dancers have long known that a low-carbohydrate, high-fat diet can improve body composition and enhance their performance.

Blue Zones: Models of Healthy Lifestyles

It has been noted that certain communities in areas known as "blue zones" have a high number of centenarians (i.e., those living to the age of 100 or longer) among them. These include the provinces of Nuoro and Ogliastra in Sardinia, Italy, which have the highest number of male centenarians in the world, the Greek island of Ikaria (popularly known as "the island where people forget to die"), Okinawa in Japan (which has 15% of the world's total number of centenarians), the Nikoya peninsula in Costa Rica and the Seventh-Day Adventist community in Loma Linda, California, USA.

Obviously, these communities then also have very low rates of chronic diseases. Yet they are linguistically, culturally, and geographically unrelated. So, what do they have in common that gives them such a remarkable level of longevity?

In all of them, the population is very physically active, either farming, walking, harvesting, shepherding, or fishing.

They are relatively small and rural or secluded, so the pace of life is considerably slower – and the level of stress commensurately lower.

They are closely-knit communities where people socialise a lot and enjoy strong emotional and recreational connections.

They have strong familial (and extended familial) bonds, where grandparents are integrally involved in the lives and care of their grandchildren. This means that the older generations are still highly active mentally and continually stimulated.

They have a strong sense of purpose and therefore lower levels of depression and mental illness.

Their diets are heart-healthy, low-calorie and include plenty of fruit, vegetables (especially beans, which are a staple food), legumes and nuts, as well as lean protein such as line-fish, with meat usually eaten only four or five times a month (and then only in small portions, as an accompaniment to – rather than the main ingredient of – a meal). Their daily portions of food are typically smaller than those of people in big urban centres. On average, they eat a meal only until they are 80% "full" – very rarely to the point of satiety or excess. Their intake of carbohydrates is high, primarily comprising wheat, oats, spelt and barley. In addition, their alcohol intake is modest, usually comprising no more than a small glass or two of red wine per day. Crucially, though, all the above communities use **olive oil** – the healthiest oil for brain health – liberally. This heart-healthy, mono-unsaturated oil has a high antioxidant level and contains polyphenols, which protect and preserve vitamin E. It is no exaggeration to say that if we could consume up to one litre of olive oil a week, we could protect ourselves from cognitive decline.

Another community renowned for its centenarians is Bama Yao in southern Guangxi, China, which is aptly named Longevity. A remote settlement, set among mountains alongside the Panyang River, it enjoys a clean environment with almost zero carbon emissions and smog. The villagers follow the traditional diet their ancestors did, comprising mainly rice, hominy (maize kernels), beans, peas, lentils, sweet potatoes, sweetcorn, fresh fruit, nuts, and seeds. Their food is prepared with hempseed oil, which is very high in polyunsaturated fats. The villagers' food is low in calories and high in carbohydrates, vitamins, minerals, and fibre.

India, too, has a low incidence of Alzheimer's disease, which has a lot to do with the fact that its population eat foods which are prepared with spices containing brain-protective properties, such as turmeric (the signature spice of Indian curries), which is a powerful antioxidant and anti-inflammatory agent. Turmeric is rich in curcumin, which helps keep neurons healthy.

Of the antioxidants, glutathione is considered the most beneficial. It is produced internally, but is also found in onions, garlic, asparagus, avocado, spinach, broccoli, cabbage, and cauliflower.

Superfoods

So, we know that certain vegetables, fruit, spices, and oils are particularly healthful and beneficial in helping to prevent the conditions that lead to cognitive decline. They include foods that contain high levels of vitamins C, E, beta-carotene, selenium, phytonutrients (such as those found in orange vegetables like carrots and sweet potatoes) and anthocyanins (which give cherries their bright red colour).

Blackberries, blueberries, citrus fruits like oranges and lemons, Brazil nuts, walnuts, dark-coloured beans, spinach, peppers, and asparagus are rich in antioxidants that help protect the brain. These are deservedly called "superfoods". Fatty fish like salmon, mackerel and herring are recommended, while sardines (especially those tinned in olive oil) are particularly nutritious, easily available in inexpensive. Just one serving of sardines provides 17g of protein, half the daily recommended amount of calcium and is rich in Omega-3 fatty acids, which help prevent inflammation.

NUTRACEUTICALS, HERBS AND SUPPLEMENTS

Nutraceuticals (natural foods, including antioxidants, dietary supplements, fortified dairy products, citrus fruits, whole coffee fruit extract (coffee berry), vitamins, minerals, herbal teas, milk, and cereals) provide trophic support to the brain. Bromelain (an enzyme derived from pineapples), methionine (an amino acid found in meat, fish, and dairy products) and chamomile all reduce histamine levels and therefore inflammation. L-glutamine (the most abundant amino acid in the body) – which is found in many foods, including sauerkraut, kimchi, miso, tempeh, yoghurt, and kefir – reduces excitability of the brain cells. Vitamin supplements (particularly vitamins B and C, which reduce histamine levels) may be prescribed. A weight loss programme may also be drawn up for the patient, including these nutraceuticals and vitamins.

Omega-3 fatty acid is essential for brain health and is also linked to cardiac health, better vision and reduced inflammatory response.

Also recommended are lion's mane (a medicinal mushroom), phosphatidylserine (a fatty substance which covers and protects every cell in the body – supplements are manufactured from cabbage and soy), phospholipids (currently produced in the form of lecithin), theanine (found in black and green tea leaves, as well as mushrooms), plenty of vegetables (including green beans), good-quality fats, oils, olives, and nuts.

Testing of hormone levels must be done before supplements are given. These tests can be expensive (in South Africa, it costs about R2 600 to test pregnenolone, for example).

Berberine – a natural isoquinoline alkaloid extracted from the traditional medical plant *Coptis chinensis* – helps to alleviate mitochondrial and synaptic damage in the brain's hippocampal neurons. This damage is caused by an accumulation of amyloid-β (a pathogenic peptide resembling a sticky compound that disrupts communication between brain cells and eventually kills them). Berberine is able to cross the blood-brain barrier, which means it can exert a beneficial neuroprotective effect against neurodegenerative agents such as homocysteic acid, calculin A, 6-hydroxydopamine, streptozotocin and mercury.

Homocysteine is made in the body from another amino acid, methionine, and plays a key role in supporting the fundamental processes upon which life depends, including preventing a multitude of illnesses such as Alzheimer's disease, cardiovascular disease, cancer, autoimmune diseases, bone density loss and stroke. However, as with many other amino acids, too much homocysteine in the system can cause oxidative stress, accelerate ageing, damage arteries, weaken the immune system, damage the brain, and impact the IQ. It can also cause blood-clotting, inflammation, pain, and lead to hormonal problems. As such, high homocysteine is a marker for many chronic health conditions and is caused by lifestyle factors including stress, poor diet, exposure to toxins and certain drugs, such as birth control pills, diabetic and antacid medications. Homocysteine levels can also increase because of an estrogen deficiency. Homocysteine levels above 76 UMOL/L have been shown to cause brain inflammation, destruction of the blood-brain barrier and weakened immune health.

In healthy individuals, methylation normally keeps homocysteine levels in check. However, for this to happen, the body needs sufficient sources of methyl from the vitamin B found in foods. It may also require supplementary sources such as Emothion (S-acetyl-glutathione), sulphated methionine (SAMe), L-5-MTHF, methylfolate, pyridox-yl-5-phosphate (P5P), methylcobalamine and Quatrefolic, the newest and best form of folic acid/folate. These convert homocysteine to glutathione, a substance produced naturally by the liver and also found in meat, fruit, and vegetables. Glutathione is essential for many processes in the body, including tissue-building and repair, making chemicals and proteins, and boosting the immune system.

Ideally, everyone – particularly those suffering from cognitive decline and the other diseases mentioned above, those with a family history of cardiovascular disease, those with premature atherosclerosis (i.e., before the age of 40), as well as strict vegetarians and vegans, who are also at higher risk of methylation impairment due to an inadequate intake of vitamin B12 – should have their homocysteine levels checked and augmented, if necessary.

HYPERBARIC OXYGEN THERAPY
Hyperbaric oxygen therapy aims to improve the circulation of blood in the body, stimulate new blood vessel growth, ameliorate atherosclerosis (the build-up of plaque on the artery walls, leading to the obstruction of blood flow) and prevent other circulatory diseases, including diabetes. It can also promote the increase and use of stem cells, reduce the risk of infection, reduce stress and anxiety, and support the immune system. It helps the brain by stimulating the

growth of new neurons, aiding neuroplasticity (the ability of neural networks in the brain to change through growth and re-organisation) and improving memory and reaction times, helps the heart by improving oxygenation to cardiac tissue, therefore reducing the risk of coronary disease, and improves heart muscle functioning after a heart attack. It assists the eyes by combatting macular degeneration, vision deterioration caused by diabetes and symptoms of glaucoma. Hyperbaric oxygen therapy is also greatly beneficial in boosting wound-healing, especially where infections do not respond to antibiotic treatment.

Moreover, hyperbaric oxygen therapy has been found to significantly reduce inflammation in the body – including the brain and the gut. Inflammation typically accompanies illnesses such as Alzheimer's disease, Parkinson's disease, autism cancer, stroke, diabetes, traumatic brain injury, irritable bowel syndrome, ulcerative colitis, osteoarthritis, rheumatoid arthritis, and tendinitis.

OZONE THERAPY

Ozone therapy helps to inactivate bacteria (by disrupting the bacterial cell envelope through oxidation of the lipids and lipoproteins). It also inactivates viruses by disrupting virus-to-cell contact through peroxidation. In addition, ozone therapy helps to inactivate fungi, yeast, and protozoa. It enhances circulation by reducing the clumping of red blood cells, thus improving oxygenation of the tissues. There is stimulation of the enzymes, which scavenge for free radicals and protect the integrity of cell walls. Moreover, ozone reacts with the unsaturated fatty acids of the lipid layer in cellular membranes, forming hydroperoxides, and it helps to dissolve malignant tumours by inhibiting their metabolism and destroying the outer layer of malignant cells.

CANNABINOIDS

The surface of the cannabis plant, where its resinous glands (trichomes) are located, contain its therapeutic components. Foremost among these is a group of 70 chemicals called cannabinoids or phytocannabinoids (CBDs), of which the best-known is the primary psychoactive one, delta-9-tetrahydrocannabinol (THC). This is the chemical which makes cannabis a mood-altering – and occasionally hallucinogenic – drug among those who smoke or eat it recreationally.

However, the plant's therapeutic properties include a powerfully analgesic one. The human brain contains receptors (molecules on the outside of cells which receive a signal to do something specific). This signal is called CB1 and the highest concentrations of these molecules are in the basal ganglia, hippocampus, and cerebellum of the brain. More recently, another type of cannabinoid receptor (endocannabinoid) was found in the macrophages (white blood cells) of the spleen, strongly suggesting that they play a role in immune function, cell proliferation, inflammation, and pain.

This, then, is why CBDs have become widely used as powerful analgesics for those suffering from chronic pain (e.g., cancer patients, chronic orthopaedic conditions, pancreatic diseases, etc). The legalisation of cannabis for this therapeutic purpose was followed by a proliferation of CBD products in pharmacies, most of them lacking the THC component, so that consumers would not "get high" off the preparation, but merely experience pain relief. However, the endocannabinoid is also believed to help prevent Alzheimer's disease and other age-related neurodegenerative disorders. The CBD's serotonin-balancing properties act as an anti-depressant, reduce anxiety and appetite, enhance sleep, and help relieve nausea and vomiting. In addition, it helps regulate blood pressure, facilitates bone re-absorptions, helps protect against methicillin resistant Strephylococcus aureus (the staph infection which commonly plagues many hospitals) and acts as a cytotoxic to breast cancer and other cancerous cells.

PHOTOBIOMODULATION

Infra-red light, directed at low levels transcranially, is useful for mitochondrial activation and has been found to assist patients with cognitive decline, as well as those with Parkinson's disease, multiple sclerosis, and motor neuron disease.

DETOXIFICATION THERAPIES TO IMPROVE COGNITION

These include glutathione drips, liposomal glutathione, infra-red saunas, and binders such as cholestyramine for mould.

UNDERSTANDING THE ROLE OF ELECTRICITY IN COGNITIVE ABILITY

There are basically four measures that determine the relationship between brain function and the creation and delivery of human electricity, which unlocks the "ageing code" and restores youthfulness, vibrancy, and health. These four measures are voltage, speed, rhythm, and synchronicity.

Voltage (Dopamine Levels)

Voltage or dopamine measures the power of electricity, i.e., the intensity with which the brain responds to a stimulus and how effectively it can process information. This information can be both cognitive and physical. The voltage is what determines the rate of metabolism and how the body processes food. It also determines a person's state of consciousness (ranging from fully alert to deep sleep) and this, in turn, determines how efficiently they are able to respond to their own emotional and physical needs, as well as those of others.

Low dopamine levels contribute to accelerated ageing by causing several "pauses" in the body:

Cardiopause, or an ageing heart, means there is raised blood pressure, weight gain, fatigue, an ageing vascular system, and high cholesterol levels.

Immunopause means that the body is unable to combat infections efficiently. If a person is obese as well, their risk of developing cancer rises substantially.

Menopause means that there is a loss of hormones, which greatly accelerates ageing.

Andropause means that a man loses genital size, as well as libido, while his risk of prostate or heart disease is heightened.

Osteopause means that fat seeps into the bones, increasing the risk of both arthritis and osteoporosis.

Dermatopause means that the skin loses elasticity, while weight gain causes stretch marks.

Hormone Treatments to Enhance Dopamine Levels

Testosterone for low sex drive; *estrogen* for ageing skin, poor circulation, menopausal symptoms, thinning hair and poor dental health; *DHEA* for fatigue; *thyroid* for depression, persistent exhaustion, and weight gain; *human growth hormone* for loss of bone mass and muscle tone, as well as ageing skin; *erythropoietin* for anaemia due for dysfunctional kidneys; *calcitonin* for bone loss; *insulin or incretin* for blood sugar regulation; *cholecystokinin* for digestive problems.

Natural Treatments to Combat Obesity

While replenishing dopamine levels is essential, it is equally important to address nutrient deficiencies and embark on an exercise regime and a proper diet to restore a lean, healthy body.

Conjugated linoleic acid, gamma-linoleic acid and 7-keto DHEA facilitate weight loss; *Garcinia cambogia* (hydroxycitric acid) with chromium suppresses appetite and inhibits the conversion of carbohydrates to fat; 5HTP reduces appetite; phenylalanine stimulates the burning of fatty tissue and increases the sensation of satiety after eating; fish oil facilitates weight loss, raises serotonin levels and decreases appetite; vitamin D, magnesium and calcium help weight loss by controlling metabolic syndrome.

Foods Which Enhance Dopamine Levels

Fruit (apples, avocado, olives, pomegranates), vegetables (broccoli, carrots, soybeans, spinach), canola oil, poultry (chicken, duck, turkey), chocolate, eggs, meat (venison, lean beef), granola, low-fat dairy products (e.g., yoghurt), fish (mackerel, salmon, tuna), oat flakes, tofu, unsalted nuts, wheatgerm.

Speed (Acetylcholine)

Speed measures the pace at which we can think or process information. Electrical signal speed in the body is governed by acetylcholine. Faster brain speed means increased attention, a higher IQ and better receptiveness to mental and social stimuli. Conversely, slow brain speed means forgetfulness, disorientation, inattentiveness, and dementia. Lack of acetylcholine to the brain means rapid ageing (osteopause, menopause, andropause and cardiopause), as well as vasculopause (leading to diabetes and vision disorders) and somatopause (increasing the risk of multiple sclerosis, memory loss and neuromuscular deterioration).

Hormones Which Promote Acetylcholine Function

Human growth hormone, vasopressin, DHEA, calcitonin and parathyroid hormone.

Nutraceuticals Which Promote Acetylcholine Function

Choline, DMAE, acetyl-L carnitine, phosphatidylserine, alpha lipoic acid, fish oils (Omega-3), GPC, manganese, CLA and piracetam.

Herbal Treatments Which Promote Acetylcholine Function

Huperzine, Vinpocetine, Gingko biloba, *Bacopa monnieri*, Gotu Kola.

Foods That Promote Acetylcholine Function

Low acetylcholine levels basically send the body a message that it is drying up. The result is a craving for fatty foods. However, Omega-3 fats are a better choice, since they boost brain speed while simultaneously breaking the fat code.

- Replace cream and whole or condensed milk with skim or non-fat milk.
- Avoid processed or smoked meat and replace it with lean beef, chicken, turkey, or fish.
- Avoid full-fat cheeses and replace them with low-fat or cottage cheese, or with low-fat yoghurt.
- Avoid ice cream.
- Replace salad dressing with low-calorie dressings, vinegar, and lemon juice.
- Replace fried eggs with boiled or poached eggs.
- Include asparagus in the regular diet.
- Increase the intake of basil, sage, salvia, black pepper, turmeric, lemon, rosemary, and mint.

Rhythm (Gamma-Aminobutyric Acid (Gaba))

Rhythm measures the balance between the two hemispheres of the brain and the flow of electrical conduction between them. The beginning of brain dysfunction is indicated by bursts of abnormal electrical activity called arrhythmias. Irregular rhythm affects one's ability to cope with stress and increases anxiety, nervousness, and irritability, as well as causing irregularities in the bowel, lungs, or joints.

Foods to Enhance Gaba
Fruit (bananas, figs, grapefruit, oranges), vegetables (broccoli, spinach, kale, potatoes), brown rice, rice bran, wholegrain breads and cereals, nuts (almonds, walnuts), meat (ox liver), fish (halibut), lentils and oats.

Hormonal Treatments to Enhance Gaba
Progesterone, pregnenolone and DHEA.

Natural Supplements to Enhance Gaba
Inositol, vitamin B3, branched-chain amino acids, taurine, glycine, magnesium, theanine, tryptophan, phenylalanine, St John's Wort.

Lifestyle Modifications to Improve Gaba Levels
Sufficient sleep, exercise (yoga), meditation, alternative therapies (acupuncture, physiotherapy), emotional support from friends and family, controlling stress levels, avoiding caffeine, and instead drinking green tea, oolong tea, white tea, or rooibos tea.

Synchronicity (Serotonin)

Synchronicity in the brain is what balances the four brain waves (alpha, beta, theta, and delta). When synchronicity is out of balance, depression, anxiety, and sleep disorders set in. Lack of sleep, in turn, triggers the cycle of inflammation. Increasing the body's levels of tryptophan through the diet can increase serotonin and augment synchronicity.

A lack of serotonin can also increase calcification in the body, leading to osteopause, lower the sex drive by lowering estrogen and progesterone levels, weaken the immune system and accelerate skin ageing, leading to loss of collagen and the appearance of wrinkles, frown lines and "crow's feet".

Foods to Enhance Serotonin

Turkey, fruit (blueberries, bananas, avocado), bran cereal, fish (salmon), dairy products (yoghurt, cottage cheese), poached eggs, tofu, and broccoli.

Herbs and Spices to Enhance Serotonin

Basil, black pepper, borage, cayenne pepper, cumin, nutmeg, peppermint, rosemary, sage, thyme, turmeric.

Hormones to Boost Serotonin

Progesterone, human growth hormone and pregnenolone.

Natural Supplements to Boost Serotonin

Melatonin, tryptophan, vitamins B3 and B6, fish oils and magnesium.

HORMONES

Synthetic Hormone Replacements

Prior to 2002, women undergoing menopause were routinely prescribed estrogen plus progestin (Provera) (i.e., synthetic progesterone plus Premarin). However, in that year, women who had not had hysterectomies and were taking these synthetic hormones were found to have an increased risk (26%) of breast cancer, as well as heart attacks.

According to a study conducted by the USA's Women's Health Initiative Programme on 16 000 women who had not had hysterectomies, and were on estrogen plus progestin, the stroke rate among them was 41% higher, the rate of blood clots was doubled, and the risk of heart disease was 22% higher. However, they were also found to have a 37% decreased risk of colorectal cancer, a 33% decreased risk of hip fractures and a 24% decreased risk of total fracture.

These findings were confirmed in additional studies, which showed that synthetic progesterone had an unfavourable effect on lipid levels and could promote cardiovascular disease.

Besides this, many women who were prescribed these synthetic hormones stopped taking them after one year because they could not tolerate their side-effects. It was found that the hormones were transmitting incomplete messages to cells, resulting in a loss of energy and an unbalanced hormonal response.

What do we make of this? On balance, it is clear that the risks posed by synthetic hormone replacements far outweigh the benefits and that patients urged by their doctors to begin such a regime (of whom there are many) should insist on an alternative treatment.

Natural Hormone Replenishment

Natural hormone replenishment (i.e., hormones which are biologically identical to those made by the body) is advised for the relief of menopausal symptoms or adrenal fatigue. They may also be beneficial in preventing memory loss and can delay the onset (and increase the risk) of cognitive decline. In addition, they can aid in preventing osteoporosis and in promoting bone growth and repair. What is more, natural hormone replenishment has been found to have no associated increased risk of cardiovascular illness.

A note of caution: Estrogen should not be administered orally, as it has been found to have a number of adverse effects. Instead, it should be given transdermally.

Natural progesterone (as opposed to the synthetic hormone progestin) offers numerous benefits. It helps balance estrogen, is quickly eliminated by the body, promotes sleep and calmness, lowers high blood pressure, helps the body use and eliminate fats, lowers cholesterol, may protect against breast cancer, increases scalp hair, normalises the libido, helps balance fluid in cells, improves the effects of estrogen on blood vessel dilation in atherosclerotic plaque, does not diminish the benefits of estrogen, increases the metabolic rate, and is a natural diuretic and anti-depressant.

Of the natural replenishments for progesterone, estriol has been found to be particularly beneficial. It does not initiate carcinogenesis (the development of cancer cells) and can help prevent mammary tumours.

Replenishing Estrogen Levels Without Hormone Supplements

This can best be done by partaking in moderate, regular exercise, eating cruciferous (crunchy) vegetables, increasing one's intake of flax, soy and lean protein, Omega-3 fatty acids, vitamins B6 and B12, folic acid and indole 3 carbinol.

Growth Hormone (GH) Replacement

In those losing GH, replacement results in a reduction in total and visceral fat and an increase in lean body mass. There is also an improvement in cardiovascular function, a reversal of atherosclerotic changes, an increase in bone density, improved cognition (memory, alertness, and concentration), enhanced sexual performance, higher energy levels, better immune function, lower blood pressure, tauter and thicker skin, a reduction in cellulite, sharper vision, and improved quality of sleep. However, GH replacement is contra-indicated in individuals with active malignancies (cancer).

Testosterone Therapy

Apart from sexual benefits, replenishing testosterone improves body composition, due to an increase in muscle. Fat is reduced and over time (up to three years of treatment), bone density is increased (particularly in the hips and spine). Higher testosterone levels reduce the risk of developing diabetes and carotid atherosclerosis in later life, while both total and LGH cholesterol levels are reduced. Men with low testosterone levels tend to have a higher mortality rate and are at greater risk of developing prostate cancer.

Testosterone therapy can be given via a number of ways:

- Injections (either short- or long-acting), typically every week or fortnight. Blood levels must be checked midway through the treatment cycle.
- Transdermal patches, depending on the degree of deficiency in a patient. There is a risk of skin irritation developing at the site of the patch.

- Orally, in pill form, although this is associated with liver toxicity. Only one form of oral testosterone – Andriol – is known not to cause hepatic problems.
- Gels (very commonly used in the USA), through which absorption tends to be better than through transdermal patches.
- Extended-release pellets inserted under the skin, typically in the buttocks. These can maintain good levels of testosterone for three to six months.
- Compounded prescriptions (creams, gels, sublingual products).
- Stimulatory medicines (clomiphene citrate and anastrozole) which "fool" the body's negative feedback, causing an increase of luteinising hormones, which stimulate testosterone. Clomiphene citrate also increases sperm counts.

The side-effects of testosterone therapy include erythrocytosis (too many red blood cells – i.e., anaemia), reduction in testicular size, acne and enlarged prostate.

Thyroid Treatment

Factors such as stress levels and stress management must be addressed. Treatment includes giving good nutritional multivitamins and additional selenium, zinc, and chromium.

INTERMITTENT FASTING

This has long been a controversial practice, with some die-ticians maintaining that no healthy, balanced diet should include periods of compete deprivation, as people tend to compensate for it by binge-eating afterwards.

However, a growing body of scientists believe that inter-mittent fasting (i.e., of solid foods, but continuing to drink fluids), in fact, has many health benefits. For one thing, it allows the body to put more energy and focus on effective immune regulation. It does this by controlling the levels of inflammatory cytokines (small groups of proteins, peptides or glycoproteins that are secreted by cells in the immune system). Two of these cytokines – Interleukin-6 and tumour necrosis factor alpha – play a particularly important role in causing inflammation in the body.

Not consuming solid foodstuffs while continuing to drink water and cleansing beverages helps flush out the digestive system and reduce the number of natural micro-organisms in the gut.

Autophagy and Fasting

Fasting also stimulates a metabolic process called *autophagy* (meaning, literally, "self-devouring" or "self-eating"), in which the body breaks down old, damaged, and abnormally developing cells and recycles them for energy – something like recycling cellular debris and "taking out the trash". An accumulation of waste, because of decreased recycling, is thought to be common to all ageing cells.

Autophagy has many longevity-boosting benefits:

- It restricts viral infections and the growth of intracellular parasites, cancer, and tumour cells. This process is part of the innate immune system and it uses special receptor to identify viral cell invaders.
- It protects the brain and tissue cells from abnormal growths, toxicity, and chronic inflammation. This means that old cellular material which is causing oxidative stress is replaced with new, rejuvenated cells by converting the worn-out cells into energy.
- It strengthens the immune system.
- It eliminates pathogens and toxins.

The Mitochondrial Theory of Ageing

According to this theory, reactive oxygen species (free radicals), which cause damage to DNA and RNA (both nucleic acids), as well as to proteins, may cause cells to die. This, of course, results in a shorter life expectancy – so autophagy is critical in preserving mitochondrial functioning and keeping the body youthful by eliminating the accumulation of free radicals.

Autophagy And mTOR

Autophagy is regulated through the pathways of the two kinases, the mammalian target of rapamycin (mTOR) and AMP-activated protein kinase (AMPK) (both encoded in genes). The one kinase, mTORm promotes *anabolism* (the set of metabolic pathways which construct molecules from smaller units – i.e., constructive metabolism), while the other kinase – AMKP – promotes the opposite process of *catabolism* (the breaking down complex molecules into simpler ones, together with the release of energy, i.e., destructive metabolism).

These two kinases have a discordant relationship: mTOR *inhibits* the autophagy process because it supports cellular growth, whereas AMPK *helps* autophagy because when a person is experiencing nutrient deprivation, AMPK blocks cellular growth, forcing the body to catabolise (break down) its weakest parts, in order to preserve the stronger, healthier ones. This sounds a lot more complicated than it actually is think of a company. When times are good and sales are high, it can afford to expand, take on new employees and venture into new areas of trade. However, when times are bad, e.g., during an economic recession, it may have to retrench employees and get rid of divisions and departments which are not part of its main area of business, in order to ensure that its core services can continue functioning. So, autophagy is really the "downsizing" component of the body.

Although autophagy is a catabolic process that involves protein breakdown, it is needed for muscle homeostasis (balance). It helps the body cope with stressors such as exercise and fasting (just as retrenchment and downsizing help a company cope with stressors such as inflation, an unfavourable exchange rate and the Covid-19 lockdown). However, *dysfunctional* autophagy contributes to ageing through sarcopenia (muscle loss). At the same time, excessive autophagy can also lead to the breakdown of lean tissue and cause muscle disorders, which can also accelerate premature ageing and make one more prone to other metabolic diseases. (To continue our metaphor, downsizing or retrenching valuable employees when times are *good* will severely impact a company's bottom line and its ability to innovate and remain competitive within in its sector.)

The entire body and all its cells are made of protein, which requires the presence of anabolic precursors and building blocks. That is why it needs mTOR and amino acids for existence and DNA repair.

The Dark Side Of mTOR Complex

mTOR is the master anabolic regulator (i.e., the trigger of cell construction) which also organises many other nutrient sensors, such as insulin, leptin, and insulin-like-growth-factor (IGF-1).

IGF-1 is a hormone that supports growth development, healing, muscle-building, and bone- strengthening. When the pituitary gland in the brain releases human growth hormone, then the liver produces IGF-1 and stimulates anabolism. However, just as a good businessman is one who can accurately read the economic climate and balance his company's production, outlay and employee complement accordingly, the body needs to achieve and maintain the correct balance for a healthy metabolism. Over-stimulation of cell growth and too-high levels of IGF-1 are associated with different types of cancers.

How to Increase Autophagy

The most effective and easiest way to promote autophagy is to do intermittent fasting (see below).

Control the insulin and blood sugar levels. Carbohydrates and amino acids from protein will suppress autophagy directly by stimulating insulin, IGF-1 and mTOR. For that reason, neither a high-carbohydrate nor a high-protein diet is advisable (or, indeed, sustainable) on a long-term basis. They should only be used for brief periods, if at all.

Restricting calorie intake and methionine restriction can decrease mTOR activity and promote life extension. Again, however, this must be done within reason, depending on one's lifestyle, age, overall condition of health and activity levels.

Exercise can also stimulate autophagy, provided it is done in a state of glycogen depletion in which AMPK has been activated. This means that it should be done before one consumes carbohydrates (i.e., before a workout or strenuous physical activity). In that way, the autophagy is activated while one is exercising, so the food one eats later is used primarily for lean muscle growth – not for storing fat or accelerating ageing.

Nutrients for Activating Autophagy

Rapamycin (an antifungal agent which inhibits mTOR and suppresses tumours), sulforaphane (found in green, leafy and crunchy vegetables, such as Brussels sprouts), curcumin, piperine (which is found in black pepper and also boosts the availability of curcumin, making it a double win!), medicinal mushrooms such as chaga, reishi, shiitake and lion's mane, ginger (containing the compound 6-Shogoal,which induces autophagy and inhibits the AKT/mTOR pathway in non-small-cell lung cancer), resveratrol (which inhibits breast cancer growth), EGCC (a compound found in green tea), Malabar tamarind, berberine, rapamycin, polyphenols and flavonoids (found in dark berries, dark leafy green vegetables and all kinds of herbs and spices).

In addition, intermittent fasting promotes the process of genetic repair, because during times of food scarcity, cells have a longer lifespan. During fasting, less energy is used to repair a cell than is used to divide and create new ones. As a result, the rapid rate at which cancer cells divide and take control of a body is slowed down.

The process of cellular (tissue) repair is controlled by the human growth hormone (HGH), which creates the metabolic changes that cause us to burn fat. While this is happening, the body uses amino acids and enzymes to improve the functions of the muscles, tendons, ligaments, and bones. Research has found that men who had fasted for 24 hours had a 2 000% increase in circulating HGH, while women had a 1 300% increase in HGH. Both men and women had significantly reduced their triglycerides, boosted their HDL cholesterol, and stabilised their blood sugar.

All of which is compelling evidence of the advantages to be gained from intermittent fasting. Ideally, one would need to fast for 16 hours a day to enter a true fasting state. However, this is neither realistic nor practicable for most people, especially those who work. So, the next-best way of undertaking it is by eating nothing for 12 hours after dinner until breakfast the next morning. This gives the body four hours to complete digestion and another eight hours for the liver to complete its detoxification. Once this has become a daily habit, one could try extending the fast one day a week for 16-18 hours and, finally, for a full 24 hours once a week, in addition to extended fasts of about three days a few times a year. **NB:** Remaining well hydrated during any length of fast is essential, provided the fluid one drinks is either water or a non-sweetened, herbal beverage.

TREATING INFECTIONS

- If detected in a patient, the herpes simplex virus type 1 (HSV1) may require a combination of an anti-inflammatory agent and olive leaf extract, colloidal silver, and lysine (found in meat, fish, dairy products, eggs, and plants such as soy and other legumes).

- Since MARCoNS is an antibiotic-resistant staph, patients who are resistant to penicillin or quinolone could be given nasal Bactroban or oral rifampicin for one to two months.

- Mould infections should be treated with binders (clay or 4g of pure cholestyramine resin taken one hour before food or two hours after meals). This may cause some bloating or constipation, especially in patients with Lyme disease. Welchol may also be prescribed (usually three measures of 625mg twice daily).

- Patients should be advised to use good-quality air purifiers in their homes or workplaces, as well as disinfect these environments regularly.

- Lyme disease must be treated quickly, as blood spread occurs rapidly after a tick bite. Steroids and immune suppressants should never be prescribed. Many patients are resistant to penicillins and cephalosporins. High doses of tetracyclines and combination treatments (e.g., with erythromycin) are often effective. In addition, the patient should get more sleep, avoid caffeine, alcohol, and nicotine, take exercise, and eat a diet high in lean protein and fibre and low in fat. Nutritional supplements should also be considered.

- Helicobacter pylori can be treated with Berberine, betaine hydrochloride, glutamine, Xylitol, Astaxanthin, melatonin, lauric acid, linoleic acid, hydrochloric acid and bile acid (both found in the digestive system), polyphenols such as catechins, curcumin, kaempferol and oleuropein, lactoferrin, whey protein and vitamins B12 and C. Certain micro-organisms may also inhibit the development of the bacteria, while smart drugs such as idebenone, sulfuric compounds, dimethyl sulfoxide and sulforaphane can help to kill it. The patient should be advised to eat bee products such as propolis and honey (only Manuka), dairy products such as bovine colostrum and yoghurt, berries (bilberries, blueberries, cranberries, elderberries, raspberries, and strawberries), red wine, olive oil, cumin seeds, grapefruit seeds and garlic. There is a wide range of pharmaceutical drugs suitable for treating Helicobacter pylori, though pharmaceutical antibiotics are not able to eradicate the infection.

- Patients with or at risk of periodontal disease may require topical or oral antibiotics. They must also be advised to undertake a strict regimen of proper dental hygiene (regular visits to dentists and oral hygienists, as well as twice-daily brushing and flossing). They should not smoke and should have the appropriate nutritional supplementation, antioxidants, grapeseed extract and CoQ10.

- Candida infections respond to antioxidants, beta carotene and Bromelain, as well as pre- and probiotics. Vitamins and minerals which help eliminate it include copper, zinc, apo-lactoferrin, co-enzyme Q10, biotin and vitamins C and E. Herbs such as black walnut, goldenseal, mastic gum, olive leaf and Pau d'arco are also recommended, as are garlic, grapefruit seed extract, coconut oil and oils made from oreganum, thyme, peppermint, rosemary, and tea tree.

TREATING CHRONIC OR SYSTEMIC ILLNESSES

- Alternative treatments for **multiple sclerosis** and other neurodegenerative diseases include avoiding fatty acids found in processed food, soy oil, canola oil and corn oil, and increasing the intake of fish oil and flaxseed oil. The patient should avoid mercury, which is a neurotoxin found in certain fish, remove dental amalgams containing mercury and consider having chelation therapy – a procedure in which a synthetic solution called EDTA (ethylenediaminetetraacetic acid) is injected into the bloodstream to remove heavy metals and minerals from the body. Glutathione may be prescribed for mercury detoxification. Vitamin D supplements should be given, as well as low-dose naltrexone, which is used to treat a wide range of auto-immune diseases and cancer malignancies. The patient should also be asked whether they suffered emotional trauma in early childhood, an event which is often associated with auto-immune diseases, and to try techniques such as meditation, prayer, and energy psychology.

- **Histapenia** (low levels of histamine caused by over-methylation) is treated by administering high levels of zinc, manganese, vitamins C and B12,

cysteine, GLA, EPA/DHA, niacinamide and querce-
tin. Patients should be put onto a high-protein diet
and avoid refined carbohydrates (white bread, pastries,
white rice, potato crisps, etc). As the copper levels
in the system are reduced, the patient's symptoms
are eased. In cases of **histadelia** (high levels of histamine caused by under-methylation), L-methionine
(an essential amino acid) and a smaller amount of
the chemical compound S-adenosyl methionine are
prescribed, as well as choline, glutathione, copper,
folate, zinc, vitamins C and B6 and calcium/magne-
sium. Since histadelic patients often experience sleep
problems, a mild sedative or sleeping pill may also
be given. Their diet should exclude vegetable oils,
processed foods, gluten, and soy, but should include
organic fresh vegetables, grass-fed beef, wild salmon,
full-fat yoghurt, and eggs.

- **Pyroluria** is treated with vitamins B6, C and E, zinc,
  manganese, niacinamide, pantothenic acid, Omega-6
  fatty acids/GLA and cysteine.

- **Vitamin B6 deficiency** can be rectified by prescribing
  up to 1 000mg of the vitamin a day, as well as zinc.
  Caution should be exercised when discontinuing treatment, as abruptly stopping a large intake of B6 can
  result in catatonia (a state of extreme unresponsiveness

to any stimuli), muscle weakness or chills with fever. Instead, withdrawal should be gradual (by 10% per day). The patient should be monitored for signs of sensory neuropathy (loss of feeling in the extremities).

Addressing a **calcium/magnesium imbalance** requires the doctor to interpret the imbalance correctly. Cortisone will lower the calcium levels, but raise both sodium and potassium levels. Lead and cadmium toxicity will displace calcium.

TREATING SLEEP DISORDERS

Patients should be encouraged to partake in mild, daily exercise, such as an evening walk for the elderly. Napping should be limited during the daytime and medications should be evaluated. The quality of light in the patient's bedroom should not be too bright, the room temperature should not be too warm or too cold, and disturbances by children, grandchildren or pets should be avoided.

A regular, relaxing routine before bedtime is a good way to establish heathy sleeping habits. The evening beverage should not contain caffeine (including soda and chocolate drinks). Alcohol and smoking should be avoided and there should be no stimulating or vigorous activities undertaken (such as watching thrillers or action movies on TV) at night; nor should there be noise or domestic arguing.

Melatonin (1-6mg, depending on age, taken 30-60 minutes before bedtime) may be prescribed. This is a potent antioxidant which also helps prevent seizures and jetlag symptoms. It should not be used during pregnancy or breastfeeding. Ideally, a course of melatonin should be short-term.

Natural/Botanical soporifics include *passionflower*, a traditional herb with sedative and anxiolytic effects, *valerian* (which hastens the onset of sleep and has been found to be at least as effective as a pharmaceutical tranquilliser) and *Rhodiola rosea* – a plant adaptogen which has been used in Russia for over 30 years to relieve environmental and climacteric stress, as well as improve physical performance in athletes. It also has cardioprotective properties and has been found to improve fatigue by up to 20% among night-shift physicians who were treated with it for three two-week periods.

Supplements which can improve sleep include 5-HTP (a precursor of serotonin, which regulates sleep, pain tolerance and carbohydrate cravings), L-tryptophan (also a precursor of serotonin), L-theanine (an amino acid found in green tea which lowers blood pressure and increases dopamine, but is non-sedating and non-addictive), magnesium (which is essential for more than 300 cellular reactions and helps relax the muscles), progesterone and, for men, testosterone, which is important for mood regulation and insomnia.

Patients who take sleeping tablets and are unable to fall asleep without them should be weaned off them carefully. Ideally, this should happen over eight weeks. For the first week, the normal dose of sleeping tablet should be taken, together with one melatonin slow-release dose. For the second and third weeks, the patient should alternate taking half a sleeping tablet one night and a full tablet the next, together with one melatonin slow-release dose every night. For the fourth and fifth weeks, the patient should take only half a sleeping tablet every night, together with one melatonin slow-release dose. For the sixth, seventh and eighth weeks, the patient should alternate taking only half a sleeping tablet one night and no tablet at all the next, but having one melatonin slow-release every night. From the beginning of the ninth week and going forward, the patient should take no more sleeping tablets at all, but continue taking one melatonin slow-release dose every night for three to six months, before stopping all medications and supplements completely.

TREATING TOXICITY

As noted previously, a high toxic burden is caused by exposure to toxins, leaky gut, yeast, bacteria, parasites, nutrient deficiencies, food allergies and mould. The symptoms of toxic burden include a general feeling of being unwell, joint and muscle pain, fatigue, persistent or recurrent headaches, skin rashes, poor tolerance of exercise – and, of course, cognitive decline.

In a healthy liver, there are two major pathways of detoxification. **Phase I** is the activation of the detoxification process, when fat-soluble toxins are introduced to the body. During **phase II,** the body's P450 enzymes neutralise and transform the fat-soluble toxins into polar molecules. These molecules are now water-soluble, so they can easily be eliminated from the body. This process – known as biotransformation – may also occur in the intestines, lungs, kidney, and skin.

Typically, toxins disposed of in this way by the liver include alcohol, nicotine, phenobarbital, sulphonamides, and steroids, as well as cruciferous vegetables, char-broiled meat, high-protein foods and nartjies. Environmental toxins such as carbon tetrachloride, exhaust fumes, paint fumes, dioxins and pesticides are also eliminated by phase I and II detoxification.

However, there are certain inhibitors of this process. Grapefruit juice, turmeric, chilli peppers, clove oil and onions are among them, as are drugs which block the secretion of stomach acid, such as benzodiazepines, antihistamines, cimetidine, ketoconazole and sulfaphenazole.

A detoxification liver test can be done in which the patient takes 200mg of caffeine upon waking. Saliva samples are then collected two and eight hours later. At bedtime,

650mg of aspirin and 650mg of acetaminophen are taken and urine samples are collected for the next 10 hours. This test shows the efficiency of phases I and II of the liver's detoxification.

A *fast phase I and a slow phase II* mean that there are toxins in the body which are not being neutralised and eliminated quickly enough, so they have time to damage cells. This is treated with supplements such as NAC, GSH, glycine, Ca-d-glucarate and co-factors.

If the liver detoxification test shows the converse situation – a *slow phase I and a fast phase II* – then the liver's primary detoxification ability is impaired. This could be due to P450 enzyme inhibitors such as H2 blockers (medicines that reduce the amount of acid produced by the cells in the lining of the stomach), birth control pills, SSRI (anti-depressant drugs), heavy metals, naringenin, anti-fungals, certain antibiotics, excess sugar, trans saturated fats and possible iron deficiency. Treatment usually involves nutritional and hepatic support from indole-3-carbinol, cruciferous vegetables, garlic, rosemary, and soy. A vitamin B6 supplement may also be necessary.

Imbalances in the liver's P450 enzymes can be addressed with tailored intervention for the patient's specific detoxification profile.

Neurodetoxification

Toxins causing nerve cell and brain damage come from a variety of environmental, personal care and lifestyle sources. These include mercury in fish, pesticides sprayed on fruit and vegetables (note that there is no such thing as a "safe" pesticide, as they all cause neurodegeneration!), aluminium in deodorants, shampoo and skincare products, lead in certain lipsticks and in walls, plumbing, paint and pipes, radio waves and electric toxins from television sets, computers, cell phones, cookware, monosodium glutamate (a flavour-enhancer used widely in tinned foods, processed meats and packeted soup powders) and aspartame (an artificial sweetening agent).

These toxins promote inflammation, which leads to brain degeneration, rapid brain ageing and cognitive decline.

The most important antioxidant used by the brain to detoxify itself is glutathione, which is also found in high concentrations in the liver. Glutathione binds to the toxins and helps make them water-soluble so that they can be excreted by the kidneys into the urine.

There are several lifestyle modifications which can be made to limit exposure to neurotoxins:

- Mercury can be removed from the diet by avoiding shark meat, swordfish, king mackerel, tilefish, halibut, and white albacore tuna – the species containing the most mercury – and instead, eating wild Pacific or Alaskan salmon, tilapia, haddock, and light tuna.

- Exposure to aluminium can be reduced by avoiding construction sites where there are lead-lined or copper plumbing pipes, repairing leaking hot water taps and avoiding ceramic dishes.

- Avoid MSG, aspartame, and hydrolysed vegetable protein (a filler and flavourant used in processed food). Always check the ingredients of food products on their labels before buying them.

- Limit exposure to electronic equipment and appliances such as television sets, computers, microwave ovens, hairdryers, power lines and electric cables. When using a cell phone, use an earphone and avoid using phone shields, as manufacturers tend to increase boost power to compensate. Do not clip a cell phone onto your body.

- Avoid damp or mouldy environments in old buildings, do not drink tap water and limit consumption of processed oils, hydrogenated fats, margarine, canola oil, mustard, peanut butter, or peanut oil, commercially made mayonnaise or salad dressings containing trans fats.

- It can be extremely beneficial to clear pathogens out of the liver, biliary tree, gallbladder, and gastro-intestinal tract by having a liver flush. This also helps heal cellular membranes.

- Glutathione is the body's major defence against toxic oxygen products. It maintains protein structure and function, stabilises the immune function, protects the body against oxidative damage and aids in detoxifying reactive chemicals. For these reasons, a glutathione intravenous push for three to five minutes relieves the body of metal toxicity and neurotoxins. The infusion should comprise 1 400mg glutathione in 9cc of sterile water, with the initial push being 1 800-2 400mg twice a week for 20 weeks. For children, the infusion should be 200-800mg twice weekly for 20 weeks.

- Curcumin (turmeric) is extremely beneficial in helping to prevent the production of tumour-producing and carcinogenic hormones. It is therefore able to enhance chemotherapy. It is a powerful antioxidant (300% more potent than vitamin E) which breaks down toxins in the liver and is also an effective anti-inflammatory.

- Resveratrol is excellent for inducing cancer cells to die off, particularly in patients undergoing chemotherapy or radiation. These treatments cause cancer cells to break open and release their contents, damaging neighbouring cells and provoking inflammation. The way cancer cells are killed may determine the severity of side-effects of cancer treatments and, indeed, the survival of cancer patients. In the body, white blood cells digest cellular debris – a process called apoptosis. Resveratrol has a powerful ability to induce this process by converting the fats in the outer membranes of tumour cells into molecules called ceramides.

The average person is likely to have 500-1 000 times higher levels of toxic chemicals in the fat compartments of their bodies (which includes fatty adipose tissues, the brain, and lipids in blood) than is revealed in their blood serum. A simple way of detoxifying is to use the lean body mass because toxins are fat-soluble and are released when the fat is burned for fuel or energy to maintain the body functions. Effective detoxification of body fat can be done using niacin (a form of vitamin B) combined with infra-red sauna therapy, exercise, and heat in order to promote sweating. Substances such as activated charcoal, zeolite clay and oils can also help to bind toxic chemicals which are then eliminated through the gastro-intestinal tract. As a measure of how effective niacin can be, Dr David Root – an American physician recognised as a leading expert in sauna-based human detoxification – worked with veteran soldiers who had been exposed to the toxic chemical Agent Orange in the Vietnam war. He successfully used niacin to mobilise fat to unlock the toxic chemical in their lipophilic fatty tissues (i.e., in their body fat and brains).

Similarly, other individuals who have been exposed to highly toxic situations – such as the fire-fighters who entered the burning Twin Towers in New York during the 9/11 attacks in 2001 – were slowly worked up to a dose of 5 000mg of niacin over the course of 30 days. Individuals who are regularly exposed to toxins (such as hairdressers who work with hair dye on a daily basis) are also advised to have high-dosage niacin detoxification.

In people exposed to lower levels of toxins, 100mg of niacin once or twice a week – followed 20 minutes later by exercise (which increases cardiac output and causes widening of the blood cells), and then a sauna or a hot bath to "sweat out" the toxins – is usually sufficient. A higher dose of niacin can induce a "niacin flush" lasting for approximately 30 minutes. Taking a cold shower can help relieve any discomfort this causes. It is advisable to start with a lower dose of about 50mg a day and, once the patient has grown accustomed to that, to work up to 100mg or more. Since sweating causes the loss of essential minerals and vitamins, it is important to replenish these with electrolytes and potassium. Coconut water is also an excellent rehydrator.

Some medical experts believe that saunas (either with or without niacin) should be a part of everyone's normal routine, if possible (ideally, twice a week after exercise), in order to prevent the build-up of toxins and inflammagens in the body.

NIACIN: A VICTIM OF BAD SCIENCE – AND BAD PRESS

Despite the body of scientific evidence attesting to the effectiveness of niacin in eliminating memory problems, detoxifying the body, and reducing inflammation, it initially met with an extraordinary body of resistance from the medical fraternity. Or perhaps the resistance was not so extraordinary after all, given the notorious conservatism and hostility of the profession – as well as the aversion of Big Pharma – to many innovations, particularly those coming from outside its narrow, accredited confines. Anyone who saw the film *Lorenzo's Oil*, or who is familiar with the story of the Odone family's battle with their 10-year-old son's adrenoleukodystrophy (ALD), will recall the knee-jerk obduracy and intransigence they encountered in the specialists, dieticians and even the support groups they turned to. ALD is a rare hereditary disease in young males which causes the build-up of very long fatty chain acids in the brain. This, in turn, destroys the protective myelin sheath around nerve cells which are responsible for brain function, resulting in progressive muscular and neural degeneration, including dysphagia, the loss of movement, co-ordination, vision, hearing, speech, bowel and bladder control. Despite the insistence of their son's doctors that nothing could be done for him or any of his fellow-sufferers (most of whom were expected to die within two years of diagnosis), Augusto and Michaela Odone embarked on their own, exhausting, self-funded quest to conduct research into the disease and find a treatment. The result was an oil comprising a 4:1 mix of oleic and erucic acid, derived from rapeseed oil and olive oil, which greatly slowed the progression of the disease and gave Lorenzo Odone another 20 years of life.

While the story of niacin is hardly this extreme, its initial reception was not dissimilar. In 2008, the use of micronutrients such as niacinamide was largely peripheral – the province of "alternative" healthcare practitioners, not to be taken seriously. Although the media announced that in a study conducted at the University of California at Irvine, "huge doses [2 000-3 000mg] of an ordinary vitamin appeared to eliminate memory problems in mice with the rodent equivalent of Alzheimer's disease", they hurriedly added that "scientists aren't ready to recommend that people try the vitamin on their own, outside of normal doses". Specifically, the study had included large amounts of nicotinamide, the vitamin B3 widely found in foods such as meat, poultry, fish, nuts, and seeds. It is also found in far greater quantities in dietary supplements. It is inexpensive and its safety has been conclusively established, apart from the possibility of nausea – a side-effect which can easily be eliminated by using regular niacin or inositol hexaniacinate instead.

Naysayers included the Chief Executive of the UK Alzheimer's Research Trust, who declared: "Until the human research is completed, people shouldn't start taking the supplement... People should be wary about changing their diet or taking supplements. In high doses, vitamin B3 can be toxic." This erroneous statement was subsequently repeated by the *Irish Times* and later endorsed by the BBC, which also cautioned: "We should even be wary about changing our diets." Fundamentalism, it seems, is alive and well and living in the world's hallowed newsrooms and broadcasting studios.

In fact, it would take 5 000-6 000mg of niacin per kilogram of body weight to kill a dog. In humans, it would take a monstrous dosage of about 375 000mg of niacin to constitute a lethal dose – and long before that amount was ingested, a person would be overcome by nausea and probably pass out or begin vomiting it up. The American Association of Poison Control Centre's Toxic Exposure Surveillance System annual reports indicate that there is not even one death a year due to niacin in any of its forms.

Why does niacin matter to patients with cognitive decline? Because there appears to be a statistically significant link between a low dietary intake of niacin and a high risk of developing Alzheimer's disease. This is not altogether surprising, since previous research has indicated that vitamins E, C and B12 may help people lower their risk of developing the condition.

The fact is that niacin and nerves go together – and nutrients are vastly safer than drugs. Orthomolecular physicians have fund niacin and other nutrients to be effective treatments for obsessive-compulsive disorder, anxiety, bipolar disorder, depression, and psychotic illnesses such as schizophrenia. When a person's brain is in danger of dying because it has not been properly fed, it is irresponsible and dangerous to delay the use of optimum nutrition.

Patricia Kane's no-amylose diet, which decreases inflammation, and her neurodetox diet are excellent strategies to prevent the onset of cognitive decline (or help reverse it once it has begun).

THE NO-AMYLOSE DIET TO DECREASE INFLAMMATION

REMOVE: All grains (wheat, rice, barley, millet, rye, and oats), all vegetables grown underground (potatoes, carrots, parsnips, beets, radishes, peanuts, onions), garlic, bananas, glucose, dextrose, sucrose, corn syrup, sugar and maltodextrin, fatty foods, soft drinks and tinned or bottled fruit juices, as well as yoghurt.

PERMITTED: Protein, milk, cheese, fresh fruit and fruit juices, all vegetables grown above ground, popcorn, tortillas, nuts, seeds, legumes, beans, and olive oil.

ADVISED: Low-carbohydrate foods, leafy greens, eggs, wild salmon, sardines, grass-fed protein sources, salads, green vegetables, essential fats, and oils.

THE NEURODETOX DIET

REMOVE: Grains (wheat, rice, barley, millet, rye, oats and corn), pasta, bread, crackers, biscuits, muffins, cereals, starchy vegetables (potatoes, carrots, parsnips, beets, radishes, rutabaga, peas), fruit (except for berries and low-carb fruits such as watermelon, cantaloupe, avocados, Honeydew melons and peaches), glucose, dextrose, sucrose, corn syrup, sugar, honey, maltodextrin, fast foods, soft drinks, sweetened yoghurts, MSG, aspartame, diet drinks, sorbitol, mannitol, maltitol, sucralose, hydrogenated vegetable oil, margarine, processed oils, canola oil, peanuts, peanut oil, mustard, mayonnaise and salad dressing.

PERMITTED: Protein at each meal (organic meat, poultry, eggs, wild salmon, sardines), raw organic seeds, nuts, organic 4:1 Omega-6 or Omega-3 rich oils, free-range organic eggs, organic butter, cream, homemade kefir with lactic acid bacteria, cold-pressed oils (e.g. sunflower, grapeseed, hempseed, safflower), oils for cooking at high temperature (butter, extra-virgin olive oil, coconut butter), soft organic cheeses (cottage, ricotta, mozzarella, goat's milk, feta), cucumbers, chives, chard, kale, cauliflower, cabbage, sprouts, celery, onions, parsley, zucchini, asparagus, broccoli, bok choy, peppers, Brussels sprouts, eggplant, green beans, tomatoes), green leafy vegetables, salads, fresh herbs and spices.

ADVISED: CA/mg butyrate twice or four times a day, Omega-6, or Omega-3 (4:1), evening primrose oil, trace minerals, ascorbic acid, organic flaxseed, chlorella, and water (not straight from a tap).

Additional supplementation
This is available for both the above diets.

Bile salts (150mg after meals containing fat), lipase containing enzymes, probiotics, vitamin D, folinic acid, methylcobalamin, carnosine, magnesium, bromelain, branched-chain amino acids, biotin, B vitamins, phosphatidylcholine, mastic gum.

TREATING MOULDS AND BIOTOXINS
Mould can damage and disable multiple organs and systems in the body, including the respiratory, haematological, immunological, and neurological systems. It is also a key cause of inhalational Alzheimer's disease and cognitive decline.

Moulds (stachybotris, aspergillus, penicillium, chaeto-mium, wallemia and others) are primarily inhaled from toxins in water-damaged buildings.

Biotoxins are associated with tick-borne microbes, such as borrelia, and co-infections like babesia, bartonella, ana-plasma and ehrlichia. These biotoxins are secreted by the liver into bile and re-absorbed by the body unless they are tagged by antibodies and eliminated. In genetically suscep-tible individuals, the antibodies are not able to do this. As a result, the biotoxins are not removed and lead to chronic stimulation of the immune system.

HLA typing (a kind of genetic test used to identify var-iations in a person's immune system) can assess the risk of a person whose innate immune system is over-stimulated in this way. Such an individual will likely be unable to clear tiny toxins and inflammagens they have inhaled from moulds and bacteria in water-damaged buildings. These moulds and inflammagens damage membranes and cause leaky gut, leaky blood brain barrier, leaky endothelium (the cellular lining of blood vessels) and leaky mitochondria.

Visual contrast testing measures one of the brain's key functions – distinguishing between finer and finer incre-ments of light versus darkness. This indicates the efficiency of the brain, especially in individuals who have high levels of biotoxins and moulds. An environmental test (the Envi-ronmental Relative Mould Index) can also be done.

Patients who have inhaled significant amounts of mould present a number of different biomarkers such as social avoidance, dehydration, frequent urination, excessive thirst, sensitivity to static electrical shocks, decreased muscle endurance, abnormal blood pressure after exercise, rapid weight gain and inability to lose weight (despite eating less and exercising more) and chronic fatigue.

Mould is treated with binders such as pure cholestyramine (after pre-treatment with Omega-3 for fewer side-effects such as gas, bloating and constipation). Welchol should also be prescribed.

A special version of a **magnetic resonance imaging (MRI) machine called 3T** can detect levels of iron deposition in the brain, making it a valuable method of identifying patients at risk of developing Alzheimer's disease. These individuals can then be given drugs called chelators, which remove excess iron from the body. Since iron can only be obtained from the foods a patient eats, they are advised to avoid any iron-enriched foods such as fortified grain products (including conventional flour) and red meat. They are also advised to drink tea and coffee with meals to reduce iron absorption, increase their intake of fresh vegetables, ensure that any supplements or vitamins they are taking do not contain iron (and keep vitamin C supplements, in particular, away from meat), as well as donate blood regularly.

GUT COMPONENTS: MITOCHONDRIAL MEDICINE

The gastro-intestinal system is one of the key focus areas in an integrative approach to cognitive decline, since ill-health of the gut is a contributor to toxic conditions that result in inflammation – including in the brain.

Prebiotics

While a great reservoir of medical knowledge has been accumulated about the role of antibiotics in treating gut infections, comparatively little is known about the equally important role played by **prebiotics.**

By definition, a prebiotic can be neither digested nor absorbed in the stomach or small intestine. It acts as a food source for a single or limited number of potentially beneficial bacteria in the large intestine. These change the microflora ecosystem in the colon, resulting in a healthier composition and improving digestion, as well as the strength and effectiveness of the immune system. In a nutshell, prebiotics are preventive, rather than curative.

Their function is to cause fermentation and produce the short-chain fatty acids (SCFAs) butyrate, proponoate and acetate. These SCFAs increase the quantities of beneficial bacteria (probiotics) in the colon, decrease the number of pathogenic micro-organisms, enhance disodium and water absorption, increase the production of metabolic energy, enhance the flow of blood to the colon, stimulate the nervous system and increase the production of the gastro-intestinal hormones.

Fructo-oligosaccharides (FOS) are prebiotics which consist of fructose and glucose molecules. They are found in foods such as asparagus, bananas, barley, rye, wheat, chicory, garlic, artichokes, leeks, and onions and increase mineral absorption, improve lipid levels, and help lower cholesterol. They are also used to treat atopic eczema and they stimulate the immune system, enhancing resistance to bacteria which produce lactic acid. In addition, they help modify the metabolism of carcinogens (cancer-causing agents). There are side-effects to FOS, depending on the dose given, such as flatulence, borborygmi (rumbling or gurgling of the gas and fluid in the intestines), bloating and abdominal discomfort. However, these decrease in time in most patients.

Lactulose is a disaccharide made from fructose and glucose. They provide all the same benefits as SCFAs, as well as inhibiting the growth of bacteria in the gut.

Colonic Foods

Colonic foods are not as specific as prebiotics in what they ferment and can promote bacteria which are either good or bad. The colonic foods which produce beneficial changes in intestinal flora include oat bran, carrots, brown rice, tea polyphenols and resistant starch.

Probiotics

These are "good" gut bacteria which are essential for maintaining mucosal and systemic immunity and improving the balance of nutrients and microbes in the intestinal tract. They promote overall digestive health by aiding the digestion and absorption of carbohydrates, producing vitamins, absorbing minerals, and eliminating toxins and keeping "bad" bacteria, yeasts, moulds, and viruses under control. Probiotics help prevent allergies and have been found to have anti-inflammatory potential and a beneficial influence on genes.

Probiotics are also beneficial in treating urinary tract infections, where spermicides and antibiotics can disrupt flora.

The reason probiotics are so important for overall optimal health is that 80% of the human immune system is located in the gastro-intestinal tract, where there should ideally be a balance of 85% "good" bacteria and 15% "bad" bacteria. In individuals experiencing stress, probiotics can help counter increases in pathogenic bacteria and the loss of bifidobacteria and lactobacillus.

In order to work efficiently, probiotics need to be able to colonise. This is a process which begins at birth, when micro-organisms such as E. coli, enterococci and streptococci enter the infant's gastro-intestinal (which has hitherto been sterile while in the womb). Further colonisation occurs during breastfeeding (as well as formula feeding), and later with complementary feeding.

As human beings age, there are changes in the bacteria which colonise the gastro-intestinal tract and vagina. By midlife, there is a significant increase in E. coli and clostridia, and a decrease in bifidobacteria. By menopause, there is a further increase in E. coli and a decrease in lactobacilli. Estrogen replacement therapy can help restore vaginal flora to the pre-menopausal state.

Some probiotics occur naturally in the human gut. They can also be found in fermented foods such as yoghurt, kefir, kombucha, sauerkraut, pickles, miso, tempeh, kimchi, sourdough bread and certain cheeses.

Probiotic supplementation may be necessary in patients with high cholesterol and triglyceride levels.

Treating Gut-Related Problems

There are basically five "R" s in this programme: remove, replace, reinoculate, repair and rebalance.

- *Remove* inflammatory foods, processed foods, and foods that you might be allergic to.
- *Replace* these with digestive enzymes, stomach acid and bile.
- *Reinoculate* good bacteria.

- *Repair* the gastro-intestinal mucosa by providing nutrients.
- *Rebalance* by following an appropriate diet and making lifestyle modifications for optimum gut health.

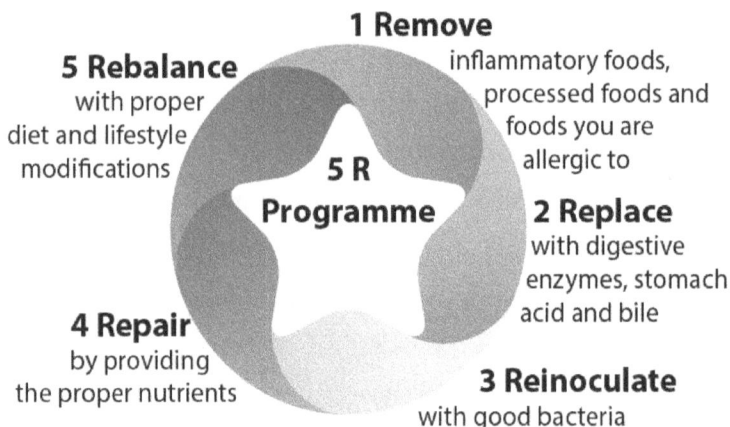

1 Remove
inflammatory foods, processed foods and foods you are allergic to

5 Rebalance
with proper diet and lifestyle modifications

5 R Programme

2 Replace
with digestive enzymes, stomach acid and bile

4 Repair
by providing the proper nutrients

3 Reinoculate
with good bacteria

THE ROLE OF NEUROACTIVE NOOTROPICS (I.E., SMART DRUGS AND COGNITIVE ENHANCERS) IN TREATMENT

Nicotinamide mononucleotide (NMN) and nicotinamide riboside (NR, an alternative form of vitamin B3) are both precursors and important pathways for the co-enzyme nicotinamide adenine dinucleotide (NAD+). (The term "precursors" can be understood as different routes, using different forms of transportation, but all leading to the same destination.) Scientists first discovered NAD+ in 1906 and since then, their understanding of its importance has continued to grow. This co-enzyme is critical for hundreds of metabolic processes, including turning nutrients into energy in a process called *cellular respiration*. This refers to the breakdown of foods such as glucose, carbohydrates, lipids, and proteins to make the energy-carrying molecule adenosine triphosphate. In cellular respiration, the extraction of energy from food molecules is called oxidation (the removal of hydrogen). This is where NAD+ is essential. It is equally crucial for the process of fermentation.

However, the human body does not have a limitless supply of NAD+. Like many other things, it declines with age.

How can it be augmented? By administering NR and NMN, which – besides being an intermediate in NAD+ biosynthesis – has also been found to play a part in preventing cardiac and cerebral ischaemia, Alzheimer's disease, diet- and age-induced Type 2 diabetes and obesity. In addition, NR and NMN are both orally bio-available and do not produce the side-effects commonly associated with other nootropics, such as hepatotoxicity (chemical-driven liver damage) or flushing of the skin.

NAD levels can also be raised by intermittent or prolonged fasting, vigorous or high-intensity exercise, taking cold showers or saunas, eating parsley, or drinking parsley juice (which prevents the destruction of NAD in the body), eating blueberries and extra-virgin olive oil, or having NAD administered intravenously from time to time. NMN is also available as an NMN/resveratrol powder mix.

Certain foods help the functioning of NAD by activating the sirtuins (proteins that rely on the presence of NAD+ to function). These include arugula, buckwheat, capers, celery, chillies, cocoa, coffee, garlic, green tea, kale, Medjool dates, red endives, red onions, red wine, soy, strawberries, turmeric, and walnuts.

THE EFFECT OF GUT BACTERIA ON THE BRAIN

Gastro-intestinal infections affect the gut-brain axis by producing amino acids (tryptophan, GABA) and chemicals (norepinephrine, 5-HT, acetylcholine) that cause neural inflammation.

MITOCHONDRIA

Although mitochondria resemble bacteria in many ways (including their double membrane and DNA structure), they are actually the power plants of cells and play a crucial role in fuel metabolism and energy production. They have their own genome and divide independently of the cell in which they reside. Mitochondria are inherited only from the maternal germ line and if they are compromised – for example, by environmental factors such as radiation, toxic chemicals, microbial imbalance, or genetic mutation – they can cause various metabolic abnormalities, most of which initially present as fatigue that is not relieved by rest.

Chronic fatigue and chronic diseases are the result of increased energy demand which the body is unable to supply. Mitochondria are vital in providing that required energy. The mitochondrial inner membrane hosts the most important vitamin conversion reactions of the cell. It converts the energy of nutrients into electrochemical potential which, in turn, drives the conversion of adenosine biphosphate (ADP) into adenosine triphosphate (ATP).

Mitochondrial dysfunction has been linked to virtually all killer diseases of ageing, from Alzheimer's disease and Type 2 diabetes to heart failure. Researchers have recorded evidence of greater mitochondrial damage in the brain cells of humans over 70 compared with those in their early 40s. In fact, many scientists believe that mitochondrial longevity determines overall longevity.

MAINTAINING MITOCHONDRIAL HEALTH: COQ10 AND PQQ

Co-enzyme Q10 (Coq10) is a compound made by the body and stored in the mitochondria of cells. Coq10 is incorporated into the mitochondria of cells, where it facilitates the transformation of fats and sugars into energy. Coq10 production decreases with age, or because of deficiencies of nutrients such as vitamin B6, genetic defects, increased demands by tissues because of disease, mitochondrial diseases, or the side-effects of treatment with statins (cho-lesterol-lowering drugs). When this happens, the ability of cells to sustain even basic metabolic functions is impaired. The result is the development of multiple disorders typical of normal ageing (including cognitive decline). However, Coq10 levels can be fully restored by taking the correct dose of supplemental Coq10.

A co-enzyme called pyrroloquinoline quinone (PQQ) has been shown to induce the growth of new mitochondria in ageing cells.

While Coq10 optimises mitochondrial function, PQQ activates genes that govern mitochondrial reproduction, protection, and repair. PQQ also provides potent protection for the heart and defence against brain degeneration.

Mitochondrial and cellular membrane damage can be reduced at four levels, by:

- Lowering exposure to environmental pollutants, with oxidising properties or free radicals.
- Increasing the levels of endogenous (internal) and exogenous (external) antioxidants.
- Lowering oxidative stress by stabilising the mitochondrial inner membranes.
- Replacing damaged membrane lipids with undamaged, polyunsaturated phospholipids.

Maintaining Mitochondrial Health

Mitochondria have their own DNA, so they are able to multiply independently of cellular division. However, it is possible to help produce new ones through the micronutrient pyrroloquinoline quinone (PQQ), which also has an extraordinary capacity to provide extra defence against mitochondrial decay – and mitochondrial decay has been linked to cognitive decline such as Alzheimer's disease, as well as to ageing, Type 2 diabetes and cardiac disease. Indeed, scientists believe that mitochondrial longevity determines overall longevity. Studies show that just 20mg of PQQ plus 300mg of CoQ10 can significantly reverse age-related cognitive decline.

PQQ also helps reduce the dangerous effect of excitotoxicity (a state in which the brain's neurons are overstimulated by toxic chemicals or electronic impulses) and protects the brain from memory-damaging plaque.

CARNITINE

Carnitine is an ammonium compound which supports energy metabolism by carrying long-chain fatty acids into the mitochondria to be oxidised for energy production. It also assists in removing products of metabolism from cells.

The acetyl-l-carnitine form is the preferred form of carnitine for cognition and brain health.

PHOTOBIOMODULATION
Intravenous Laser Therapy

There are specific cells in the body which are able to absorb particular wavelengths (colours) of light (called photoreceptors). The light sends a cellular signal which affects the behaviour of chemicals, the metabolism, movement, and gene expression. This means that all the body's enzymes and proteins are affected across entire cells, including the mitochondria.

Red laser has a positive influence on the flow of blood throughout the body, stimulates the immune system, improves the supply of oxygen to tissue, helps develop "giant mitochondria" by activating various metabolic pathways, has a sedative effect and helps with pain relief. It also stimulates the functional activity of the hypothalamus in the brain and the limbic system.

Green laser binds to haemoglobin, improves the function, behaviour, and elasticity of red blood cells, increases oxygen delivery, and improves blood flow.

Blue laser helps with vasodilatation and with growth, the immune system and neural functioning. It stimulates stem cell proliferation and plays a critical role in pain relief, vasodilation, and cardiac health. It lowers blood pressure and is also an anti-inflammagen. In addition, blue light is used to treat infections and it releases *nitric oxide*, which has multiple benefits, including:

- Increasing energy production
- Increasing blood flow to vital organs
- Boosting exercise performance and endurance
- Managing diabetes by regulating insulin
- Lowering blood pressure and "bad" cholesterol
- Reversing the formation of atherosclerotic plaque
- Reversing kidney failure and renal disease
- Improving sexual performance
- Offsetting damage caused by nicotine
- Enhancing memory and cognitive function.

Yellow laser improves the antioxidant enzyme and hormone systems and has a detoxifying effect. It also has strong anti-depressant effects, especially when combined with hypericin (found in St John's Wort), and helps with pain relief, mood stabilisation and vitamin D production.

Ultraviolet light increases the absorption of oxygen into body tissues, destroys fungal, viral, and bacterial growth, improves blood circulation by dilating blood vessels, improves the body's ability to detoxify, stimulates the production of vitamin D and restores the normal size and movement of fat elements.

Transcranial Low-Level Laser Therapy and The Led Infrared Helmet

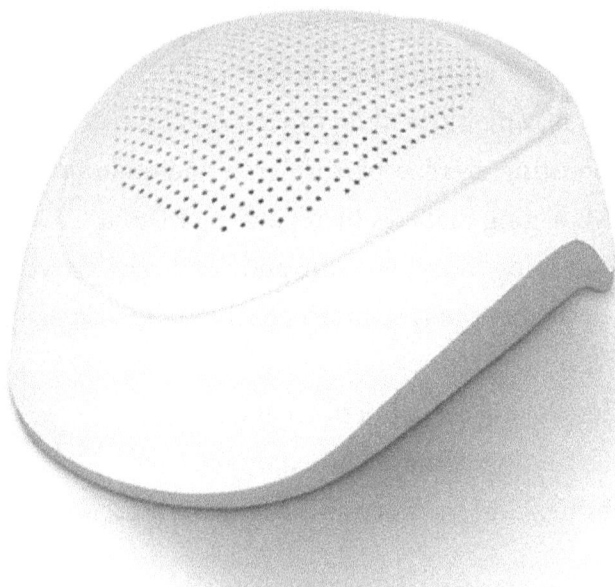

The use of transcranial (i.e., passing through the skull) light has become increasingly popular in treating neurodegenerative diseases, including Alzheimer's and Parkinson's diseases. It is also being used increasingly to treat depression, strokes, and post-trauma brain injuries.

How does it work? By stimulating the mitochondrial respiratory chain, thus releasing nitrous oxide, improving oxygen availability and consumption, activating long-lasting changes in protein expression, improving lymphatic flow, stimulating adenosine triphosphate production, helping the brain repair itself and protecting it from inflammation and excitotoxicity.

Daily transcranial low-level light laser treatments lasting about 30 minutes are generally recommended for optimum results, as patients can now purchase their own LED infrared helmets at a cost of €2 900-3 200 (about R52 700-60 000 as at March 2021). The frequency of the light ranges from 1-20 000Hz.

The ideal wavelength for maximum skull penetration is 805-830nm (infrared), with the light reaching a depth of 4-5cm. The treatments are non-invasive, non-thermal and painless.

D-RIBOSE

The role played by D-ribose – a critically important sugar molecule believed by some to improve exercise performance – in cardiovascular health was first noted by two American cardiologists, Drs Stephen Sinatra, and James Roberts, when they began adding it to the Coq10 and carnitine which they were giving their patients. Once these patients began taking D-ribose, the doctors noticed an astonishing drop in their hospital admissions.

D-ribose is now being widely used to prevent and reverse cardiovascular disease before catastrophe strikes. Every cell in the human body uses D-ribose, but to varying degrees and slowly. It is produced mostly in the liver, adrenal glands, and fat tissue. The heart, skeletal muscles, brain, and nerve tissue only produce enough of it for their daily needs. Red meat (especially veal) contains the highest dietary concentration of D-ribose, but still not enough to provide meaningful nutritional support to patients with cardiovascular disease. These patients must take D-ribose in supplementary form every day, as missing even one day can impact cellular energy and result in weakness and fatigue. Different dosages are advised for different conditions. As a starting point, 5g (or two teaspoons of it in powder form) should be given for cardiovascular prevention, to healthy people doing strenuous activity and to athletes on maintenance. 10-15g daily should be given to patients with heart failure or other forms of cardiovascular disease, as well as those recovering from heart surgery or heart attacks, those suffering from stable angina and athletes working out with chronic bouts of high-intensity exercise. Patients with advanced heart failure, frequent angina, those awaiting heart transplants and those with fibromyalgia or neuromuscular disease should be given 15-30g of D-ribose daily.

TREATING PARKINSON'S DISEASE

As with other neurodegenerative diseases like Alzheimer's disease, multiple sclerosis and motor neuron disease, an integrative approach is required to treatment. This means assessing the patient's medical profile, lifestyle, and environment, as well as providing supplementary nutrients.

Low-dose naltrexone (i.e., 3-4,5mg at night) will elevate the endorphins, which orchestrate the activity of stem cells, natural killer cells, and other immune cells. Transcranial LED infrared light is also showing very promising results in treating both Parkinson's and Alzheimer's.

Glutathione – which is often lacking in Parkinson's patients – is crucial in managing their condition. It helps to preserve brain tissue by preventing damage from free radicals. It also recycles vitamins C and E, further preventing brain tissue damage, and has the unique ability to make the brain more sensitive to dopamine. However, care must be taken to avoid giving them acetaminophen or Panado, as this can further reduce liver glutathione.

It is also necessary to detoxify certain chemicals and metals to which Parkinson's patients have been exposed, including pesticides, herbicides, aluminium and mercury, since it has been found that there is a flaw in their ability to detoxify themselves. Alpha lipoic acid is not only an antioxidant, but a metal chelator, while gingko biloba is extremely useful in detoxifying herbicides and other chemical agents.

Emothion is the nutrient of choice for these patients, as it contains orally absorbable glutathione. Levodopa (L-dopa), also known as l-3,4-dihydroxyphenylalanine – an amino acid produced and used in normal human biology – is also essential to address the inability of Parkinson's patients' brain to produce dopamine, while nicotinamide adenine dinucleotide (NADH) has yielded encouraging results in improving their condition. Since Parkinson's patients also lack co-enzyme Q-10 (especially in those taking statin drugs), they should be given ubiquinol. Phosphatidylserine can help enhance the effectiveness of what little dopamine remains, while vitamins C and E have been shown to extend the time until patients require L-dopa by a median of 2,2 years. In addition, acetyl-L-carnitine increases energy production in damaged neurons.

Remember also to support Dopamine synthesis with L-tyrosine, B6, zinc and iron when required and Omega 3 (DHA omega 3 makes up to 80% of the dopaminergic system)

Other characteristics of Parkinson's are the gut microbiome, particularly certain sensory cells in which Lewy's bodies (misfolded α-synuclein proteins) are found. It has been postulated that these misfolded proteins then travel from the gut to the brain, where they accumulate. Dr Daniel Johnstone, a scientist and researcher at the Bosch Institute of the University of Sydney, Australia, has found that exposure to infrared light alters the gut microbiome in mice – an exciting discovery, which may indicate that the same treatment in humans with Parkinson's disease (as well as other inflammatory, neurodegenerative illnesses) will yield significant improvements.

Measuring
Cognitive Decline

THERE HAVE BEEN VARIOUS tests devised over the years to assess the level of cognitive decline. Initially, these were mostly a set of standard tasks (e.g., counting backwards, being asked to draw the hands on a watch to indicate a specific time, memorising a short list of items, etc). Truly little, if any, attention was paid to the patient's metabolic functioning and, sadly, many thousands of them were labelled as "dysfunctional" and their families advised to engage home help to care for them until such time as they could be institutionalised in a geriatric facility.

Nowadays, physicians like Dale Bredesen encourage men to have a "cognoscopy" by the time they are 50 and women to have it before menopause, typically in their mid- to late 40s. A cognoscopy detects early metabolic and hormonal imbalances which are markers for Alzheimer's so that these can be rectified to prevent the onset of the disease. It involves a set of blood tests, a series of simple, online cognitive assessments and an MRI scan with volumetrics (optional, but strongly recommended for those whose cognitive scores suggest impairment).

Mini-mental and Montreal cognitive assessment testing are also used to estimate the level of cognitive decline.

However, a BRAIN ELECTRICAL ACTIVITY MAPPING (BEAM) SCAN is the most reliable test of brain function. It assesses the brain's electronic transmission by measuring four individual brain waves and brain wave combinations. It gives a graphic depiction of the four major primary brain biochemicals. The voltage determines brain power. Gamma aminobutyric acid (GABA) is a naturally occurring amino acid that works as a neurotransmitter in the brain. Neurotransmitters function as chemical messengers. GABA is considered an inhibitory neurotransmitter because it blocks, or inhibits, certain brain signals and decreases activity in the nervous system. In a BEAM scan, GABA is reflected by a measure of the brain's rhythm. A BEAM scan also determines brain speed (measured in P300 – the higher the P300, the slower the brain), reflecting acetylcholine levels, while wave balance (a reflection of serotonin activity) reflects synchronicity of the brain.

These highly technical terms may sound bewildering, but they are essentially measures of the level of heathy functioning in the brain, which tells the neurologist how severe or advanced the patient's condition is on the Alzheimer's spectrum. This – together with the information gathered about the patient's lifestyle, medical history, genetic profile, age and sleeping habits – enables the neurologist to compile a multi-pronged treatment regimen for the patient and monitor their progress, going forward.

It is crucial to remember that the amyloid plaque which has formed between neurons in the brain and disrupted cell functions is not the cause of Alzheimer's disease: it is the brain's protection against major metabolic and toxic disturbances. (Most patients manifest 10-25 of the "36 holes in the roof" caused (or exacerbated) by genetic, hormonal, environmental, dietary or lifestyle factors, so classification of them is essential.) The neurologist must find and address the causes for the plaque before dissolving it.

As the biochemistry of the patient deteriorates, so does their cognition.

KEEP GOING

Therapies must be used for a lengthy time (usually about six months) to achieve significant changes in the condition, so it is important that the patient and neurologist do not give up prematurely. Even the most modest sign of improvement is an excellent indication of continued improvement to come. If the progression stops, then it is a sign that something has been missed, or that the patient may not be complying with the prescribed treatment. In this case, the neurologist needs to review the causes of the patient's condition and make the appropriate changes. It is necessary to continually evaluate, plugging "holes", addressing all the contributors to the disease, changing the patient's diet, exercise and ensuring that they take the correct supplements, hormones, and nutraceuticals.

It is also necessary to continue encouraging the patient and their family to persevere with the treatment programme.

BRAIN EXERCISES TO HELP PREVENT COGNITIVE DECLINE

An active, stimulated brain is one of the strongest defences against cognitive decline. Mental exercise is also a natural stimulant, especially for the elderly or people suffering from depression, loneliness, or anxiety.

The key is to provide mental stimulation which is enjoyable and easily available. Reading is always an excellent way of maintaining mental alertness, especially in a book club where the literature can be discussed and shared with others. Crossword puzzles, Sudoku, lectures, and adult education classes are also recommended. Playing with children or pets and taking regular exercise (walking, swimming, yoga, Pilates, gardening, etc) are excellent not only for the brain, but for the body.

There are also apps available to provide brain exercises, such as Brain Trainer, while programs like Dakim contain specially formulated brain exercises.

These activities stimulate not only the mind, but the emotions – key factors in cognitive decline.

Music (either listening, singing, or playing an instrument) is not only enjoyable, but an immensely powerful and profound source of stimulation. Famed English neurologist and writer Oliver Sacks – who did extensive research on the impact of music on patients with cognitive decline – reported that in his visits to patients in various institutions, "some of them are confused, some are agitated, some are lethargic, some have almost lost language – but all of them, without exception, respond to music".

In his books *Musicophilia: Tales of Music and the Brain* (Vintage) – about the uniquely human and healing power of music) and *The Man Who Mistook His Wife for a Hat* (Pan Macmillan – about the far reaches of neurological experience), Sacks explained that there was no single music centre in the brain, but rather 20-30 networks spread throughout it which analysed different components of music, from pitch and rhythm to melody. He also documented cases of patients who suffered comas after traumatic head injuries and, upon regaining consciousness, found that although they had previously had only limited exposure to, liking for or knowledge of music, were suddenly compelled to begin learning a music instrument and showed remarkable aptitude for it.

Afterword

THE BRAIN IS A much more resilient and regenerative organ than medicine has assumed for the past 200 years. Equally, its relationship with all other organs and systems in the human body has been vastly underestimated. Whereas previously, the very mention of the word "brain disease" struck dismay in people, we now know that it can be nourished, stimulated, and nurtured and that the support it draws from what we eat, what we inhale, how we live, how we sleep, how we move, how we work and how we play can effect miraculous recovery.

In this book, we have tried to present a "user's manual" for the brain and bring hope and new understanding to those battling with cognitive decline. We offer a very divergent approach to this because we have seen traditional medical treatments try – and fail – to address the true pathology of the condition. Our holistic modality is based on years of research, observation, and success. What we have learnt from it convinces us that we have found the correct, multi-pronged solution – on the correct scale – to a multi-pronged problem.

It is our privilege to share it with you.

Resources

Amen, Daniel G. Memory Rescue: Supercharge Your Brain, Reverse Memory Loss and Remember What Matters Most (Tyndale Momentum).

Bains, J, *et al.* "Neurodegenerative Disorders in Humans: The Role of Glutathione in Oxidative Stress-Mediated Neuronal Death", *Brain Research Reviews* 1997; 25(3):335-338.

Berger, F, Lau, C, Dahlmann, M and Ziegler, M. "Subcellular Compartmentation and Differential Catalytic Properties of the Three Human Nicotinamide Mononucleotide Adenylyltransferase Isoforms", *Journal of Biological Chemistry* 2005; 280:36334-36341 doi 10.1074/jbc.M508660200 [PubMed] [CrossRef] [Google Scholar].

Biaganowski, P and Brenner, C. "Discoveries of Nicotinamide Riboside as a Nutrient and Conserved NRK Genes Establish a Preiss-Handler Independent Route to NAD+ in Fungi and Humans", *Cell* 2004:117:495-502, doi: 10:1016/S0092-8674(04)16-7. [PubMed] (CrossRef) [Google Scholar].

Birkmayer, J, *et al.* "Nicotinamide Adenine Dinucleotide (NADH) – A New Therapeutic Approach to Parkinson's Disease: Comparison of Oral and Parenteral Application", *Acta Neurologica Scandinavica* 1993; 87(146):32-35.

Bowthorpe, Janie A. *Stop the Thyroid Madness* (Laughing Grape).

Braverman, Eric R. *Younger You* (McGraw-Hill Education).

Bredesen, Dale E. The End of Alzheimer's: The First Program to Prevent and Reverse Cognitive Decline (Avery).

Chowanadisai, W, *et al.* "Pyrroloquinoline Quinone Stimulates Mitochondrial Biogenesis Through cAMP Response Element-Binding Protein Phosphorylation and Increased PGC-1 Alpha Expression", *Journal of Biological Chemistry* 2010; 285:142-152.

Clarke, R and Stansbie, D. "Assessment of Homocysteine as a Cardiovascular Risk Factor in Clinical Practice", Review. *Annals of Clinical Biochemistry* 2001; 38:624-632.

Classen, DC, Pestotnik, SL, Evans, RS, Lloyd, JF and Burke, JP. "Adverse Drug Events in Hospitalised Patients: Excess Length of Stay, Extra Costs and Attributable Mortality", *Journal of the American Medical Association.* 1997, January 22-29; 277(4):301-306.

DiNicolantonio, James J and Mercola, Joseph. Superfuel: Ketogenic Keys to Unlock the Secrets of Good Fats, Bad Fats and Great Health (Penguin Random House).

Dotika, Randy. "Vitamin Holds Promise for Alzheimer's Disease", *HealthDay Reporter*, 5 November, 2008, http://www. washingtonpost.com/wp-dyn/content/article/2008/11/05/ AR2008110502796.html, http://health/yahoo.com/news/ healthday/vitaminholdspromiseforalzheimersdisease.html.

Evans, RJ, Derkach, V and Surprenant, A. "ATP Mediates Fast Synaptic Transmission in Mammalian Neurons", *Nature*, Vol 357, No 6 387, pp503-505, 1992. View at: Publisher Site | Google Scholar.

Foster, Harold D. *What Really Causes Alzheimer's Disease* (Trafford), 2004, ISBN 1-4120-4921-0.

Goepp, J. "Reverse Mitochondrial Damage: Potent Molecular Energisers for Lifelong Health", *Life Extension* magazine, February 2010.

Graham, D *et al.* "Oxidative Pathways for Catecholamines in the Genesis of Neuromelanin and Cytotoxic Quinones", *Molecular Pharmacology*, 1978; 14:633-643.

Green, KN, Steffan, JS, Martinez-Coria, H, Sun, X, Schreiber, SS, Thompson, LM and LaFerla, FM. "Nicotinamide Restores Recognition in Alzheimer's Disease Transgenic Mice Via a Mechanism Involving Sirtuin Inhibition and Selective Reduction of Thr231-Phosphotau", *Journal of Neuroscience*. 2006, November 5; 28:11 500-11 510.

Hauptmann, S, Scherping, I, Dröse, S, *et al.* "Mitochondrial Dysfunction: An Early Event in Alzheimer Pathology Accumulates With Age in AD Transgenic Mice", *Neurobiology of Ageing*, Vol 30, No 10, pp1 574-1 586m 2009. View at: Publisher Site | Google Scholar.

He, K, *et al.* "Antioxidant and Pro-Oxidant Properties of Pyrroloquinoline Quinone (PQQ): Implications for its Function in Biological Systems", *Biochemical Pharmacology* 2003; 65(1)67-74.

Hoffer, A and Foster, Harold D. *Feel Better, Live Longer With Vitamin B3: Nutrient Deficiency and Dependency* (CCNM Press), 2007. ISBN-10: 1897025246; ISBN-13: 978-18970252246.

Huang, N, Sorci, L, Zhang, X, Brautigam, CA, Li, X, Raffaelli, N, Magni, G, Grishin, NV, Osterman, AL and Zhang, H. "Bifunctional NMN Adenylyltransferase/ADP-Ribose Pyrophosphatase: Structure and Function in Bacterial NAD Metabolism", *Structure* 2008; 16:196-209 doi 10:1016/j.str.2007.11.017. [PMC free article] [PubMed] [CrossRef] [Google Scholar].

Mills, KF, Yoshida, S, Stein, LR, Grozio, A, Kubota, S, Sasaki, Y, Redpath P, Migaud, ME, Apte, RS, Uchida K, *et al.* "Long-Term Administration of Nicotinamide Mononucleotide Mitigates Age-Associated Physiological Decline in Mice", *Cell Metabolism* 2016; 24:795-806 doi 10:1016/j.cmet.2016.09.013. [PMC free article] [PubMed] {CrossRef] [Google Scholar].

Mosconi, Lisa. Brain Food: The Surprising Science of Eating for Cognitive Power (Avery).

Perlmutter, David. Brain Maker: The Power of Gut Microbes to Heal and Protect Your Brain (Little, Brown Spark).

Perlmutter, David. Grain Brain: The Surprising Truth About Wheat, Carbs and Sugar – Your Brain's Silent Killers (Little, Brown Spark).

Perry, T, *et al.* "Parkinson's Disease: A Disorder Due to Nigral Glutathione Deficiency", *Neuroscience Letters*, 1982; 33:305.

Pieczenik, SR and Neustad, J. "Mitochondrial Dysfunction and Molecular Pathways of Disease", *Experimental and Molecular Pathology*, 2007; 83(1):84-92.

Pozueta, J, Lefort, R and Shelanski, ML. "Synaptic Changes in Alzheimer's Disease and its Models", *Neuroscience*, Vol 251, No 5, pp51-65. 2013. View at: Publisher Site | Google Scholar.

PubChem Nicotinamide Mononucleotide/C11H15N2O8P – PubChem. Available online: https://pubchem.ncbi.nlm.nih. gov/compound/nicotinamide_mononucleotide.

Rasmussen, K and Moller, J. "Total Homocysteine Measurement in Clinical Practice", Review. *Annals of Clinical Biochemistry*, 2000; 37: 627-648.

Reddy, PH, Tripathi, R, Troung, Q, *et al.* "Abnormal Mitochondrial Dynamics and Synaptic Degeneration as Early Events in Alzheimer's Disease: Implications to Mitochondria-Targeted Antioxidant Therapeutics", *Biochimica et Biophysica Acta (BBA) – Molecular Basis of Disease*, Vol 1 822, No 55, pp639-649, 2012. View at: Publisher Site | Google Scholar.

Refsum, H, *et al.* "Facts and Recommendations About Total Homocysteine Determinations: An Expert Opinion", Review. *Clinical Chemistry*, 2004; 50(1):3-32.

Ryan, TJ and Grant, SJ. "The Origin and Evolution of Synapses", *Nature Reviews Neuroscience*, Vol 10, No 10, pp701-712, 2009. View at: Publisher Site | Google Scholar.

Sapolsky, Robert M. *Why Zebras Don't Get Ulcers* (Holt).

Sechi, G, *et al.* "Reduced Glutathione in the Treatment of Early Parkinson's Disease", *Progress in Neuro-Psychopharmacology & Biological Psychiatry*, 1996; 20(7)1 159-1 170.

Smith, Pamela Wartian. What You Must Know About Memory Loss and How You Can Stop It: A Guide to Proven Techniques and Supplements to Maintain, Strengthen or Regain Memory (Square One).

Stites, TE, *et al.* "Physiological Importance of Quinoenzymes and the Q-Quinone Family of Cofactors", *Journal of Nutrition*, 2000; 130(4):719-727.

Welch, GN and Loscalzo, J. "Homocysteine and Atherothrombosis". Review. *New England Journal of Medicine*, 1998; 338(15): 1 042-1 050.

Wilson, James L. Adrenal Fatigue: The 21st-Century Stress Syndrome (Smart Publications).

Further references available upon request.

www.ingramcontent.com/pod-product-compliance
Lightning Source LLC
Chambersburg PA
CBHW021558210326
41599CB00010B/496